I0100519

Rural Health Provisioning

Aderemi Suleiman Ajala

Rural Health Provisioning

Socio-cultural Factors Influencing Maternal
and Child Health Care in Osun State, Nigeria

PETER LANG

Frankfurt am Main · Berlin · Bern · Bruxelles · New York · Oxford · Wien

Bibliographic Information published by the Deutsche Nationalbibliothek
The Deutsche Nationalbibliothek lists this publication in the Deutsche Nationalbibliografie; detailed bibliographic data is available in the internet at http://dnb.d-nb.de.

ISBN 978-3-631-59023-2

© Peter Lang GmbH
Internationaler Verlag der Wissenschaften
Frankfurt am Main 2009
All rights reserved.

www.peterlang.de

To all my respondents who sacrificed their time for interview.

Acknowledgement

I am profoundly grateful to the institutions and people that were instrumental to this publication. The efforts of peer reviewers were acknowledged. More importantly, I appreciate the supports and cooperation enjoyed from my family, my research assistants and all my respondents during the fieldwork. My doctoral research enjoyed funding from the Centre for Legal, Social and Policy Research (CLSPR), Ottawa, Canada; that granted me a research fellowship in 2000 and the University of Ibadan postgraduate school, Nigeria that also granted me the MKO Abiola postgraduate research fellowship, 2001. CODESRIA should also be mentioned due to many of its programmes which I enjoyed during the course of my doctoral research and after (2001-2005). I am therefore very grateful to all these agencies. During the final collation, formatting and editing (2008-2009), I was a research fellow of Alexander von Humboldt Foundation (AvH), Bonn, Germany. I appreciate all these opportunities.

Foreword

Rural communities especially in many sub-Saharan Africa are characterized by higher prevalence of HIV/AIDS, malaria incidence and maternal and child morbidity and mortality among others. They as well lack enough access to healthcare facilities, while many of their health attitudes also constitute health risks. Most of the problems causing these health problems are cultural, thus, suggesting that ethnography needs be involved to understand the perspective of rural health care system. It is on this that Aderemi Suleiman Ajala made his contribution to knowledge.

Being a product of doctoral research, the book examines the conceptualization of health and illness among the rural Yoruba communities of western Nigeria. It also explains cultural attitudes that influence rural health care system. As the book specifically focuses on maternal and child health care system in six selected rural communities of Osun state, within a specific culture context, it projected into general health issues bothering rural community of Nigeria.

The author's concern on resilience of maternal and child healthcare problems and the practice of traditional medicine in rural Yoruba community of western Nigeria, transcends theoretical exposition. The author engaged in an intensive fieldwork in the study area within a period of eighteen months and empirically valid and objective data emerged on rural health provisioning. Thus, the book is of great value and predicated on well- researched data. The analysis and presentation of data as contained in the book are lucid and well-described with the conclusions deriving logically from firmly established premises. The practical relevance of the book is not also in doubt as it presents what, to all intents and purposes, amounts to a veritable template of thoughts and prognoses on the strategies for delivering rural community of sub-Saharan Africa from quagmire of maternal and child morbidity and mortality using Osun State in Nigeria as a model. These solutions are development-focused and people-friendly.

I therefore warmly recommend this book to everyone who seeks a better understanding of the nature of health care provisioning in rural community of sub-Saharan Africa, and to policy practitioners desirous of a workable policy framework for improving rural health care system. Specifically this book holds a strong promise for scholarship as it remains a recommendable text in both sociology and anthropology.

Innocent V.O. Modo (Ph.D)
Professor of Anthropology
Department of Sociology and Anthropology
University of Uyo
Uyo. Nigeria. August 2008.

Preface

This book evolved from my doctoral research held between 1999 and 2002 at Department of Sociology, University of Ibadan, Nigeria. The dissertation was supervised by Professor E.A Oke, and the ethnographic fieldwork was conducted in six selected rural communities of Osun state between 2000 and 2001. The dissertation was awarded a pre-doctoral research grants by Centre for Legal, Social and Policy Research, Ontario; and Programme for Alternative Technology in Health (PATH). Following the encouragements from these bodies and other colleagues in support of publishing the dissertation, I went back to the field between 2007 and 2008 to update my data.

The primary focus of the book is on the persistent high occurrence of maternal and child morbidity and mortality especially in sub-Saharan African societies, reflecting that much ground is yet to be covered in maternal and child healthcare, especially in the rural communities of this region. Despite the facts that health problems associated with these sectors of population are largely preventable, the attention is still directed towards curative approach, hence the resilience of high maternal and infant mortality and morbidity. The persistence of the problems further suggests that there is little understanding of social and cultural factors associated with the utilization of maternal and child healthcare (MCH) services especially in the rural communities where the severity of the problem is more apparent. The book therefore discusses socio-cultural factors influencing the utilization of MCH in the rural communities of Osun State, Nigeria with the aims of providing information on: people's conception and knowledge of MCH; how some social variables such as age, literacy level, religious and beliefs affect the practice of MCH in the research area; and examining certain traditional practices and behaviours which are either harmful or promotive to MCH in these rural communities. It also evaluates and assesses the influence of some MCH programmes in Osun State; and identified various ways of enhancing the activities of various institutions responsible for MCH, so as to drastically reduce the rate of maternal and child morbidity and mortality.

A significant part of this book is devoted to the conceptual framework, which rest on synthesis of Innovation Adoption Theory, Social Impact Assessment Model and Health Belief Model in order to theorize the background factors undermining the introduction and implementation of new health programmes and policies. Ethnographic methodology used in data collection is a triangulation of Non-participatory observation, key-informant interview and structured interview in its data collection approach.

The specific findings show that illiteracy and low level of economic activities suffered by mothers were the major causes of MCH problems. Similarly, certain harmful traditional practices such as food taboos, forced-hand feeding, teenage pregnancy and the use of traditional mixtures of herbs dominated the child health. It was also found that prolonged breast feeding, the availability of fresh fruits and vegetables are promotive to MCH. These were cultural practices being revisited and promoted.

Finally, it is concluded that the harmful attitudes and practices stated above must be discouraged and those attitudes that are promotive must be encouraged. Level of literacy also needs to be raised. Government also needs to support informal economy, speed up rural development programmes and direct poverty alleviation policies and programmes to the rural people so as to reduce maternal and infant morbidity and mortality in the rural areas. Hence, going by its contents, the book is going to be useful for scholarship.

Aderemi Suleiman Ajala
Mainz,
Germany 2009.

Acronyms

BHSS: Basic Health and Social Services Schemes.
CAC: Christ Apostolic Church.
CLSPR: Centre for Legal, Social and Policy Research.
CODESRIA: Centre for Development and Social research in Africa.
CSDR: Child Survival and Development Resolution.
EPI: Expanded Programmes on Immunization.
GOBI-FFF: Growth Monitoring Oral Rehydration therapy, Breastfeeding and Immunization, Food Supplements, Family spacing and Female education.
HBM: Health Belief Model.
LDC: Less Industrialized States.
LGAS: Local Government Areas.
MCH: Maternal and Child Health.
MCHDP: Maternal and Child Healthcare Development Programmes.
MKO: Moshood Kasimowo Olawale.
NGOs: Non-Governmental Organizations.
ORT: Oral Rehydration Therapy.
PATH: Programmes for Alternative Technology in Health.
PHC: Primary Health Care.
R&D: Research and Development.
RFH: Reproductive and Family Healthcare.
SIA: Social Impact Assessment.
SMI: Safe Motherhood Initiative.
TM: Traditional Medicine.
UNDP: United Nations Development Programmes.
UNICEF: United Nations Children's Education Funds.
UPN: Unity Party of Nigeria.
WHO: World Health Organization.
WM: Western Medicine.

Contents

1 Introduction 1
Theoretical and Conceptual Framework... 7
    Culture Change Theory.. 8
    Innovation Adoption Theory 11
    Social Impact Assessment Model... 12
    Health Belief Model (HBM).. 13
Rural as a Concept 16

2 Research Methodology and Design... 19
Methodology.. 19
The Study Population 19
Rationale for the Choice of the Study Site.. 20
Pretest... 20
Sampling Procedures 21
Method of Data Collection... 21
    Key-Informant Interview 22
    Observational Technique... 22
    Structured Interview... 23
Data management and Analysis.. 24
Ethnographic information about the study area.. 25
    Socio-linguistic Features... 25
    Residential Unit.. 26
    Political Organization 27
    Economic Activities.. 28
    Belief System.. 29
    Family... 29
Selection of Research Sites.. 30
Ethnography of the Research Sites 31
Ajaba... 31
    Political Organization... 32
    Socio-Economic Development.. 33
    Cultural Attitudes Related to Health Care... 33
    Residential Pattern... 34
Ekusa 34
    Economic Activities.. 35
    Political Organization... 35
    Socio-Economic Development.. 35
    Belief System Associated with Health Care 36
Ibodi.. 36

Socio-Economic Development... 36
Political Organization... 37
Residential Pattern.. 37
Okinni.. 37
Economic Activities.. 38
Political Organization... 39
Socio-economic Development 40
Health Behaviour and Attitude... 40
Telemu.. 41
Political Structure 42
Economic Activities.. 42
Infrastructural Development 43
Tonkere 43
Political Organization... 43
Economic Activities.. 44
Infrastructural Development in Tonkere... 44
Demographic Characteristics of the Respondents.................................. 45

3 Culture and Health... 47
Introduction... 47
Medicine and Culture 47
Traditional Medicine and Social Change 48
Maternal Child Healthcare in Nigeria 49
Cultural Factors in MCH 52

4 Knowledge and Beliefs in MCH... 53
Introduction... 53
Conception of MCH.. 53
Belief System in MCH 56

5 Social and Economic Factors in MCH 61
Customs and Habits Associated with MCH 61
Poverty and Its Effects on MCH... 65
Women Social Roles and Effects on MCH... 67

6 Rural Health Care and MCH in Osun state 69

7 Conclusion 73
Policy Implications of the Study... 76

Bibiliography.. 79

Index 87

List of Tables and Figures

Table 1: Demographic characteristics of the respondents   46
Table 2: Methods of caring in MCH in rural communities of Osun State   58
Table 3: Utilization patterns of traditional medicine in MCH   59
Table 4: Age at childbirth 65

Figure 1: Culture contents   9
Figure 2: Social and cultural variables influencing utilization of MCH
    services   15
Figure 3: Causes of maternal and child health morbidity and mortality in
    rural communities of Osun state, Nigeria   73

1

Introduction

Maternal and child healthcare system is an important segment of medical system in every society. This is as a result of large number of human population involves in this health sector, coupled with the significance of this population to the overall sustenance of any human society, as it mainly involves both women and children. Despite the fact that this sector of medical system is affected by less difficult health problems, which are usually preventable, yet it remains one of the major health problems attracting higher prevalence of morbidity and mortality especially in rural communities of sub-Saharan Africa. Thus, maternal and child health has attracted attentions, probably more than any other health sectors in the region.

Similarly, the increasing wave of gender equality has significantly stimulated attentions towards the study of women and children. It is in the light of the above that this sector has attracted overwhelming attentions especially from health related researchers, health providers and health policy implementers (Jinadu, 1998; Smyke, 1991; Royston and Armstrong, 1989). Specifically, writers have exposed the risks of childbearing and child healthcare in their various writings and research findings. The works of Jinadu (1998), Smyke (1991), Royston et. al. (1998), Richard (1974), Nevarro (1974), Odebiyi (1977 and 1999), Aregbeyen (1991), Ebrahim (1982), Owumi (1989 and 1996), Iyun (1987 and 1994) and Oke (1987, 1993 and 1996) are very significant in this respect. All these works and the annual reports of World Health Organization (WHO) and UNICEF since 1970s show that there is high maternal and child morbidity and mortality especially in Nigerian rural communities.

As observed in all cultures, each society has its peculiar ways of dealing with bio-cultural problems affecting its human population. Responses to various interventions seem to differ considering the peculiar knowledge displayed by the population in each society. Environmental factors also play considerable role on the health seeking strategies, thereby making the health interventions and responses greatly different across the culture (Richard 1974; Nevarro 1974; Odebiyi 1977).

It is noted that maternal and child healthcare problems require a preventive approach (Aregbeyen 1991; Ebrahim 1982), hence it is considered very easy to arrest. As noted above especially by Richard (1974), each culture has a peculiar way of dealing with bio-cultural problems with differing responses; sincerely responses to these problems are not the same across the culture. In industrialized countries of the world, an appreciable success has been attained in reduction of morbidity and mortality affecting the lives of both the mothers and the children (Price 1994). Whereas in less-industrialized countries of the world, despite all the attempts to reduce the severity of maternal and child healthcare (MCH) problems, it still remains a scourge which continues to claim the lives of a large percentage of their populations (Price 1994). No doubt, it still remains a major curious topic especially to behavioral scientists dealing with socio-cultural aspects of medicine (Erinosho 1998). As at 2008, health statistical indexes have shown that maternal and child morbidity and mortality is greater in less industrialized countries than what is obtained in industrialized countries of the world. For instance, infant mortality is indicated to be between 0.3%-0.6% in Finland, Sweden, Britain and United States of America, comparable with 12%-14.5% infant mortality occurring in Nigeria, Haiti, Sierra Leone and Zaire (UNICEF 1994, 1995, 1996; WHO 1991, 1992, 2008).

However, among the Yorubas of western Nigeria, especially in Yoruba rural communities, the traditional knowledge of maternal and child healthcare system is still largely upheld. In this society, MCH problems are explained through natural and preter-natural explanations. The belief in traditional practice is that diseases are sorts of punishment. Hence, health solution is in favor of appeasing gods through libations and other related rituals. The people also appease witches to get rid of their powers of snatching children from their mothers. Sometimes however, some of these health problems are adamant because gods, witches and other associated spirits refuse libations and appeasement. Hence, the traditional practices of maternal and child healthcare system featured tieing charms, amulets and bangles on mothers and children to immunize them against the wrath of gods and spirits. Yet all these attempts did not avail the Yoruba society of the security against infant and maternal morbidity and mortality. Diseases such as cholera, malaria and malnutrition often resulted in convulsions which eventually claim lives of many children usually the under fives (U-5) (Jinadu 1998). Thus in many occasions, there are many children born into a family that are claimed to be òbóbánje or Àbíkú[1] and passed away into earth beyond between age 0 and 5 (Fadipe 1970; Daramola and Aina 1967; Soyinka 1982; Clark 1981).

Upon the introduction of orthodox medicine into Yoruba society and diffusion of western scientific beliefs, knowledge and practices of modern medicine were witnessed. Although this new approach finds it difficult to finally extinguish the traditional medical approach, yet its prominence and preference is ascertainable in the urban communities, hence, leaving the rural communities to either traditional option, or plural medical care system. In this wise, the rural communities have the traditional medical system more utilized than the modern medicine. According to Aregbeyen (1992), Pearce (1978), Odebiyi (1977) and Owumi (1993), almost 75% of Nigerian population living in the rural communi-

---

1   Among the Yorubas of western Nigeria, "*Ogbanje*" or "*Abiku*" is regarded as sprit that often possessed children either in pregnancy or/and at birth and usually cause the children to die. The belief is that when a child is possessed with the spirit, there is no amount of healthcare given to such a child that can stop the child from dyeing at infancy.

ties utilize either traditional medical system singly or blend the provisions in both modern medicine and traditional medicine.

Over the years, despite the fact that the rural health care survives on either exclusive traditional health care system or the plural system, maternal and child health care problems still remain increasing. Thus, western medicine introduced some health care development programmes to avert the crises. Mainly these programmes were initiated through bilateral international and national agencies, and Non-Government Organizations (NGOs) in the areas of maternal and child healthcare system in rural communities of Nigeria, but still maternal and child health system still remains the major health problem in rural communities of western Nigeria like many other parts of Nigeria. The introduced health care development programmes included establishment of more hospitals, importation of drugs and provision of more trained medical personnel in the rural communities. Also specific maternal and child health programmes were initiated, such as the enunciation of Basic Health Services Scheme (BHSS) and Primary Health Care (PHC) System with emphasis on breastfeeding campaign. Also introduced were health promotion strategies such as health education and provision of infrastructures, yet mortality rates associated with preventable maternal and childhood diseases seem unabated (Jinadu 1998; Young 1981; Williams Bausmalang et. al. 1989).

In line with the above, it is probable that many Nigerians especially indigenes and residents of rural communities born within forty to fifty years ago might have managed to escape infant mortality by slim chances. During that time only few Nigerians survived to adulthood, while on the average fifteen pregnancies for a Nigerian woman would produce seven normal deliveries. These seven normal deliveries from a mother would avail her only three children surviving to adulthood. Cumulatively, on every 1000 children born with success, 150 of them might be committed to mother earth within three to five years of their births. No fewer than one thousand mothers out of 100,000 often lost their lives at childbirth (Jinadu 1998; WHO 1960; Population Bureau Bulletin 1999).

Some of the children that managed to survive were at one time or the other products of malnutrition, stunted growth and wasting. They regularly lived at the instance of many preventable diseases. The rural health ecology was too disturbing to the overall health development. This situation was partly due to exclusive reliance on traditional system of MCH, which failed to cope with various controllable infectious diseases, affecting the teeming population of both women and children. These diseases included cholera, marasmus, typhoid, tetanus and poliomyelitis. Diphtheria, diarrhea and measles also claim several lives of the under fives (Jinadu 1998; Ebrahim 1982; Williams Bausmalang et al 1989). Mothers too were not spared of these dreadful conditions. They suffered complications at childbirth, hemorrhage and the likes as a result of inadequate modern knowledge of motherhood. This situation in no doubt posed severe inhibitions against individual development as well as national development (Lewis 1994; Clarke 1990; Raikes 1989).

In traditional rural societies, the survival of this important segment of the population (mothers and children) was not handled with levity. Traditional Birth Attendants/pediatricians (TBA), *eléwé-omo* and the herbalists have become prominent in the intervention approach (Owumi 1993; Odebiyi 1977). Although the traditional healthcare system then was accessible, triable and affordable, yet it could not solve the problem associated with maternal and child health in these communities (Owumi 1993). It was upon this that colonialism gained ground and subsequently embarked on westernization of health care system in these societies (Schram 1971). In the 1920s, when a maternity was established in Ilesa, Osun State, it seemed that a new ground to tackle maternal and child health problems was discovered, but this hope remains unascertained. In these societies, names like *Málomó, Igbékòyí* and *Ajítòní* imply the recurrent infant mortality through the spirit of *Àbíkú* (Soyinka 1982). Even as at 2009, with the development in modern medicine as shown in establishment of complex healthcare facilities, specialized training of medical doctors and other personnel, importation of drugs and provision of modern healthcare knowledge coupled with multisectoral approaches at finding a lasting solution to infant and maternal health care problem, the plight of mothers and children still seems insecured mostly in the rural communities. Hence, comparing the rural health care profiles in Nigeria with other western societies, a great difference is reflected against Nigeria success in western medicine.

The works of Bonsi (1982); Owumi (1993); Oke (1995); Pearce (1986) and Odebiyi (1977) have specifically talked on traditional healthcare systems in different parts of African societies. Owumi (1993) and Odebiyi (1977) have studied *eléwé-omo* that is traditional pediatricians in Yoruba society of Nigeria and announced it to be meeting the health requirements of vast majority of people. Their position was that there is a need for integration of these traditional healthcare practices with orthodox system if the utility and potency in traditional medicine is to be useful to mankind.

Pearce also in 1986 distinctively noted that culture change witnessed in African societies has displaced the values of traditional system of various healthcare practices. While corroborating this assertion, Aregbeyen (1991) and Erinosho (1998) in their studies respectively observed that maternal and child healthcare systems are worst for this change. Hence, it was noticed in 1995 in another study particularly carried out in Osun State that the rural people in this State are seriously affected by imbalances introduced by the trends of change in their healthcare system (Ajala 1995, 1999).

Other writers like Williams Bausmalang and Jellife (1989), Iyun (1994), Odebiyi (1977), Oke (1993), WHO (1998), Smyke (1991) and Price (1994) have particularly observed that the need is opened to study particular socio-cultural factors responsible for the resilience and high prevalence of maternal and infant morbidity and mortality in the rural communities of less industrialized countries. It is true however that there are paucity of facts on the influence of culture on the health and ill-health of the people, yet various works in existence seem not to have found clues to the problems of maternal and child morbidity and mortality especially in rural communities of Nigeria.

The recent health profiles confirm that out of 14.8 million people who go into demise annually as at 1998, 75-80% of these are from rural communities of less developed states (LDS). 45-50% of these are mothers and children in the third world societies (WHO 1998; WHO 1996; Population Data Sheet 1997). Health indications further revealed that prior 1960, infant mortality rate in sub-Saharan Africa was 257 deaths per 1000 live births. In 1960s, it was reduced to 145 deaths per 1000 live births; while between 1980s and early 1990s, the rate oscillated between 120 deaths – 110 deaths in every 1000 live births in Nigeria. Still between 1993 and 1999 when the country faced serious economic decline and political instabilities coupled with attendant harsh micro-economic policies infant mortality rate increased to 130 deaths per 1000 live births. All these affected under five children (WHO Annual Reports 1960-1998; UNICEF Annual Report 1965-1999). Rural communities are mostly affected by all these occurrences. From the death records in developed societies, there is high rate of significant reduction of infant mortality. For instance, in Sweden, Finland and France, it was reduced from 17.0% to 3.7% between 1960 and 1985, and since 1985 to the time of writing, the reduction was to 0.6 or 0.7% in these countries. Authors attributed this decline to the activities of PHC in those countries (Penny Price 1995). Despite the establishment of PHC also in Nigeria since 1985, why is MCH problems still remain resilient?

Solution to the existing problems transcends just importation of western ideas to secure mothers and children from the scourge of preventable diseases particularly in the rural communities of Osun State. In this society there is a gravery of poor maternal and child healthcare system, reflected in infants' malnutrition, poverty, poor infrastructural facilities to support health system, and lack of dependable economic system to avail the population an access to western healthcare facilities located in distant towns and cities. These again are the obvious causes of untimely deaths of large number of mothers and children. In view of these, some who might have escaped death are not strong enough to fall into the scope of a healthy person.

Having perceived this resilient silent crisis covers socio-cultural factors influencing the utilization of maternal and child healthcare services in Nigerian rural communities taking Osun State as a study sample. The principal intention is to establish a holistic knowledge towards understanding of maternal and infant mortality and morbidity in Nigeria. This work therefore examines the effect of education, traditional knowledge and practices among the population on childbearing and childrearing practices in the study population. The research also examines the effects of micro-economic policies and available infrastructural facilities to sustain healthcare development programmes on maternal and child healthcare in the rural communities.

It considered that local customs, beliefs and certain traditional practices have effect on the success of maternal and child healthcare (MCH) programmes in rural communities. Furthermore, it also analyses various intervention strategies which have been instituted against maternal and infant mortality and morbidity and their impacts on the society.

The scope covers the examination of MCH between 1980 and 2008. MCH is phased into Traditional Methods (TM) of MCH and Western Methods (WM) of MCH for the purpose of careful examination on the changes associated with MCH over the time. MCH development programmes such as Primary Health Care (PHC) services, which incorporated Breastfeeding Campaign, Family Planning Campaign, Immunization and Health Education Strategies were carefully assessed.

This study emanated from my earlier study on cultural practices related to breastfeeding and their implications on Maternal and Child Healthcare system among the people of Ilobu, Osun State. This study on breastfeeding was conducted as Master's degree thesis in Medical Anthropology at the Institute of African Studies, University of Ibadan, Ibadan in 1995. In that study, it was discovered that despite the establishment of various maternal and child healthcare programmes and services, most rural people are still reluctant to utilize them or not utilizing them properly. Such services include family planning programmes, health education, safe motherhood initiatives, and immunization programmes among others. Non-utilization of these programmes were responsible for maternal and child morbidity and mortality in the area. Thus, following the commencement of doctoral research programme in the same University, I therefore decided to further my research on rural health provisioning, focusing on maternal and child healthcare in Osun state. This work is therefore a detail report of my doctoral research thesis focusing on socio-cultural factors affecting the utilization of maternal and child healthcare services in rural communities of Nigeria. It is a model of health care situation in Less Developed Countries (LDCs) of the world taking Osun State as a case study.

This study falls within a time-frame of 1980 up till 2008. This period is phased into three stages. The first is between 1980 and 1990 covering the period when Nigeria had just started the Second Republic; and when Nigeria first took foreign loan from International Monetary Funds. That implies that it was the time Nigeria acceded to Structural Adjustment Porgrammes, which the thesis establishes that have rippling effects on national healthcare system (Ajala 1999).

The second phase is between 1990 and 2000, when Primary Health Care (PHC) was vigorously pursued under military regimes of General Ibrahim Ba-

bangida as the Head of State and Dr. Olikoye Ransome-Kuti as the Honorable Minister of Health in Nigeria. This period saw the vigorous pursuit of PHC principles and practices. It is noted that Osun State was selected as one of the pilot studies for the commencement of PHC in Nigeria then.

The third phase is between 2000 and 2007 when the country entered into democracy under Chief Olusegun Obasanjo, who was the Nigerian president between 1999 and 2007, having firstly ruled the country as a Military head of state between 1976 and 1979. Following the initial severe economic depression and harsh micro-economic policies which the country experienced under the dictatorial government of Late General Sanni Abacha, subsidies on oil and agricultural inputs were removed and government abandoned the maintenance of infrastructural facilities at that time. More dreadful at that time was neglect of PHC programmes, and low commitment of the government to pursue Research and Development (RD) which could have yielded information on people's health profile. Frauds and corruption were the order of the day at that time, and the International community, due to political turmoil in Nigeria, began to treat the country with hostility and harshness especially on debt-servicing of the country. This study examined the effects of these experiences on the MCH system in the rural communities of Osun State. The study examines the habits, customs, beliefs and other cultural practices of the people as related to MCH in the past; juxtapose them with what they were between 1980 and 2000. Then bring out their effects on the MCH utilization pattern of services in the rural communities of Osun State.

This particular work therefore contributes to the research of others on one hand, by taking up from where they stopped. On the other, it opens a distinctive focus on anthropological study of rural healthcare development. The work investigates the present problems associated with maternal and child morbidity and mortality in the rural communities. Such scope is neglected in the existing work as a result of time constraint. These distinctions therefore make the work very relevant to subsequent researchers on culture and health development in rural communities. It is also relevant to health workers, policy makers and policy implementers of health programmes.

On the theoretical plane, the work employs multi-theoretical and multi-conceptual approaches in the analysis and investigation of its subject-matter, serving as a lasting legacy in the field of anthropology. The work specifically contributes to the potential significance of anthropological principles to solve real and practical problems affecting rural communities of Yoruba society.

Theoretical and Conceptual Framework

The study derived its theoretical strength from social change theory and underlying conceptual frameworks of rural healthcare development. Focus on social change is on Innovation and Social Impact Assessment theories. The study also uses Health Belief Model (HBM) to examine people's perception of illness, as well as conditions determining taking particular health clues in maternal and child healthcare in rural communities of Osun State.

Culture Change Theory

It is a consensus among the behavioral scientists that no society is static. According to Raymond Firth (1958: 149) the "bony structure", i.e. the basic underlying principles that give a culture form and meaning may not be easily altered but the "flesh and blood"- the traits and complexes that fill out the cultural configuration can and do change quite rapidly. Thus, healthcare system, which is an aspect of culture, similarly undergoes changes from time to time. In this wise, explanation of maternal and child healthcare emanates from social change theory. Analysis of social and behavioral change in maternal and child healthcare (MCH) reflects the causes of change, adoption of changing traits and assessment of the impacts of such changes on the population studied. In this context, innovation and its adoption is capable of explaining the changing patterns of MCH in rural communities of Osun state, western Nigeria.

Various definitions of culture ascertain that every human society has a distinctive culture which controls the behavior of its members. These cultural patterns are relative to their physical and socio-cultural environments (Oke 1987: 193). This assumption has made anthropologists to classify culture as modern and traditional, relying on the resilience and adaptive tendencies in some cultural traits. Cultural traits that are resilient are mostly referred to as traditional cultures, while the newly introduced cultural traits are referred to as modern cultures. It should be noted that the fact that there are certain cultural traits usually refer to as traditional does not imply that such aspect of culture is static. Apparently, all cultural traits do experience transformation from what they were in the past to new forms. When such transformation occurs, the beliefs and philosophy attached to such practices too are bound to adapt to the new forms.

Social change theory primarily explains the differences in attitudes, behaviours, technology or social institutions in comparison with what they were in the past. Social change involves the development of new patterns in all variables of life; which can either be synchronic or diachronic. This is to say that there are two methods of studying social change. That is synchronic and/or diachronic, thus social change assumes cultural stability and cultural change. Synchronism emphasizes culture resilience and adoption while diachronism holds to culture change as an evidence of lapse of time. However, studies tend to focus more on diachronic, but as warned by Oke (1987: 194), studying social change should not view synchronism and diachronism as mutually exclusive, rather stability and change should be considered as essential aspects of any culture of a living people. Furthermore, Linton (1945) suggested that instead of examining culture change in terms of synchronic or diachronic, a scheme for the description of culture content can be followed. He enumerated three main categories which include universals, specialties and alternatives. These three culture contents depict three concentric circles showing universals in the core zone, with the specialties making up the intermediate zone and the alternatives at the very outer zone. Linton (1945) further specifies that universal culture elements include ideas, habits and conditioned emotional responses, which are applicable to all normal adult members of a society. Specialties are those elements shared by the members of certain socially recognized groups who are distinctive categories of individuals. The total populations do not share such elements. The alternatives are those traits which are well known to all adults but with respect to which there is a free choice. Desirably, changes are more frequent in the zone of alternatives than either of the two layers. In actual fact, the universal zone seems more resilient but not static. This analysis is indicated in figure 1 below.

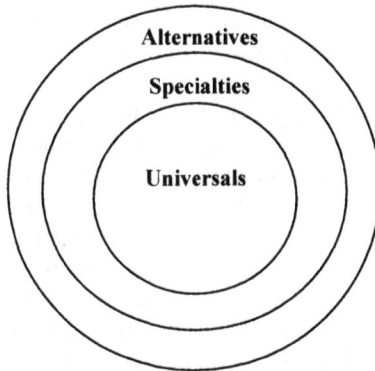

Fig 1: Culture Contents (Source: Linton's Examination of Culture)

However, as the classification of culture content fails to explain the forms of culture change and why some planned changes are often ignored, one therefore tends to associate more with Barnett in his work published in 1953. Barnett (1953) maintains that the major basis for culture change in any society is innovation. Innovation is the occurrence of new traits possible as a result of discovery or invention. In his analysis of innovations in six different cultures, he noted that innovation may occur within a particular society or by virtue of intersocietal contact or through diffusion. This simply suggests that innovation can either be endogenous or exogenous or both.

Innovation is the process of acculturation and integration. Acculturation is a change which occurs in a culture or subcultures. This process occurs when members of a cultural system have contacts with a usually more powerful group. It entails extensive borrowing in form of superordinate-subordinate relations.

External pressures in terms of information network, diplomacy and warfare usually from more powerful group are exerted on less-powerful group, and the less-powerful group assimilates the more powerful cultural traits.

Acculturation is a complex phenomenon which depends partly on the size of the population involved and the media power, the adaptability and the flexibility exhibited by the culture involved. Notably acculturation can lead to accommodation or fusion or pluralism. On the other hand, integration is the process of mutual adjustment especially when the innovation made is compatible with the pre-existing practices. This is often referred to as progressive adjustment which results to modification. It is clear that there cannot be integration without modification. In essence, it is a condition for the acceptance of innovation. In short, the concept of integration is concerned with the process of interaction which is more of what happens to the host culture during the process. Effect of this interaction may be in three folds namely replacement, alternative and syncretism.

Replacement involves extinction of one trait for the newly introduced trait, while alternative depicts the two traits co-existing while either of the two serves as alternative to other. Syncretism is blending, that is, accommodation of the two elements into one form.

From the above analysis, what is germane to our discussion here is the application of the above to changes in medical sector in Nigeria and in particular the maternal and child healthcare system in rural communities of Osun State. Changes in maternal and child healthcare in Osun State can be better analysed within synchronic and diachronic perspectives. Before the advent of colonialism, the practice was traditional which featured indigenous practices, such as long-term breast-feeding, the use of concoction and local herbs; and the patronage of traditional healers. Traditional birth attendants undertook child delivery and women were faced with numerous cultural prejudices, which posited threat to their healthcare system. Patriarchy and male-child preference principally associated with Yoruba social relationship also had effects on maternal and child healthcare in the Yoruba communities. All the above are the synchronic aspects of maternal and child healthcare which still seem resilient among the people.

The advent of colonialism, and the subsequent independence and internationalization of culture exposed the Yoruba communities to new health culture. The new health culture featured specialized training of personnel in maternal and child healthcare, nationalization and globalization of health policy and the introduction of exogenous innovations in healthcare management. Such newly introduced health cultures include modern health institutions, primary healthcare and other Maternal and Child Healthcare Development Programmes (MCHDP). All these are aimed at reducing the morbidity and mortality grossly affecting mothers and their children. Despite all these diachronic elements in MCH development, certain traditional practices are still impossible to replace. Such include the belief and practices associated with *abiku* – child mortality; high patronage and confidence in traditional therapeutic options; the practice of polygyny and preference for male-children, which are indications of patriarchy. A careful analysis of MCH development therefore depicts some resilient cultural practices such as the use of local herbs and concoction and the practice of traditional medicine as a common culture among the Yorubas. These culture contents to a large extent dominate and were given boost by socio-economic conditions of the people. The use of baby food, midwifery and immunization are the specialties which changes have brought into the MCH culture contents. Individuals too are left with the option as to either rely on western healthcare system or traditional healthcare system.

The above analysis reflects the effects of these socio-cultural changes, showing on one side, replacement and alternative; and on the other there is syncretism. Replacement occurs where certain traditional practices have gone into extinction for new practices; the alternative favors the presence of both traditional and modern practices co-existing and syncretism shows the accommodation of the two practices. All these are the features of MCH in the modern context.

Authors have noted that the effects of changes have not yielded desired development in maternal and child healthcare system in Nigeria (Odebiyi 1977; Jinadu 1998; Jegede 1998). They are of the opinions that introduction of western medicine which refuses to accommodate and integrate traditional medicine portends a great danger to a sustainable MCH development. This problem as noted by Tella (1992) is not unconnected with the process of innovations, which can be better analysed in maternal and child healthcare in rural communities of Nigeria.

Innovation Adoption Theory

Considering the problems of integration of modern medicine (MM) with the traditional medicine (TM) as well as the chance of adopting the newly introduced traits, we need to examine innovation adoption theory. Innovation as noted above is a set of new ideas, knowledge, practices and object. It encompasses specific constructs, cultural codes and forms of management and co-operation. Its adoption reflects the workings of various processes affecting the actions of individuals (Feder et. al. 1993: 256; Saginga 1998).

In consideration of the above therefore, our focus on innovation adoption theory relies on three basic factors necessary for the adoption of new healthcare programmes. These factors are:

1) Socio-economic characteristics of the adopters, which include age, education, family size, income, risk and uncertainty, belief system etc.
2) Structural and institutional factors such as information availability, policy intervention, contact, infrastructural facilities, locational factors and culture contexts etc.

3) Technological characteristics, as perceived by individuals, which include relative advantage, compatibility, complexity, triability and observability.

All the above indicated factors have effects on the utilization of new healthcare development programmes. It is evidenced from this study that the process of innovation fails to take into consideration the above factors. The above analysis provides explanation on why innovation failed to have positive impact on health care development in the rural communities of Osun state. However there are certain impacts associated with the changes in the healthcare development in rural communities of Osun state.

Social Impact Assessment Model

To describe and analyze the real impact or potential effects of health development programmes upon specific groups of peoples, we need to identify the groups of people that are affected, the distributional effects and the differential impacts of such development programmes on different categories of people. In doing this, we employed social impact assessment framework. Social Impact Assessment (SIA) is a broad concept applied to studies on social and cultural impact of development plans and programmes as well as projects (Carley and Derow 1998). It provides information on the socio-economic impacts which are associated with a new project, policy and programmes. It emphasizes the impacts of alterations on the living conditions which include changes in community patterns of life; such changes include productions, distributions and consumptions of goods and services (Campbell 1990). Thus, SIA is concerned with impact analysis focusing on how far the programme has been successful in meeting social and environmental objectives as well as appropriateness of the programmes. That is, to measure how the improved health development programmes equate with the needs and priorities of household and other units in the target population. This implies looking at the improved health technologies from the viewpoint of the users; i.e. both male and female members of the households, actual and potential and examine their social features.

From the above, it is clear that in the rural communities where western education is too low, the family size is too large with low income level, rural health provisioning is faced with a lot of uncertainties and risks. These reflected in their conception of health, by the rural people and their belief on western medicine. As their conception and perception of modern health care system is negative; the adoption of planned changes in health care system becomes problematic. Complicating the situation is the lack of positive means of health education that could have positively changed the people's conception and perception towards adoption in the rural communities. This suggests that basic information about planned change is a necessary condition for innovation adoption.

Although in some places, information was provided, yet such information is very limited and not available to vast majority of the people. Also the available infrastructural facilities could not merge the requirements of western medicine and in some cases the locations of health institutions are too remote to the users. Similarly, the attitudes of health workers in most cases are non-receptive to the health users. All these accounted for the failure of innovation in maternal and child healthcare system. In view of these factors, individuals feel that technologies associated with modern medicine do not have relative advantage because they seem to be too complex. They are therefore non-compatible, non-observable and non-triable to the rural communities.

To measure the level of utilization of rural healthcare services, there is need to examine the health decision-making of the rural people. To this end, the most appropriate theory that can explain health decision of the rural people is Health Belief Model (HBM) associated with Rosenstock (1966).

Health Belief Model (HBM)

HBM assumes that beliefs and attitudes of people are important determinants of their health related actions. The model accounts that when strategies for actions, such as assumptions are present, there can still be variations in health care utilization behavior. These variations can be explained by beliefs concerning four sets of variables. These are:

1) individual perception of his own vulnerability to illness;
2) the belief about the severity of the illness which may be defined in terms of physical harm or interference with social functioning;
3) the person's perception of the benefits associated with actions to reduce the level of severity or vulnerability; and
4) the evaluation of potential obstacles associated with the proposed actions. These actions may be physical, psychological or financial (Oluwadare 2000; Jegede 1998; Rosenstock 1966).

In essence, there must be a belief that there is intervention in disease and that the intervention would produce the desired result. Also there is a consideration for the benefit, costs and inconveniences involved in seeking a particular healthcare service.

This model therefore generates two broad actions in health care seeking, which are:

1) health seeking behaviour; and
2) decision-making process.

In decision-making process, for somebody to remain healthy, he must take positive step and act upon them. Decision-making is dependent on three other factors:

1) human nature;
2) culture; and

3) human nurture and pattern of learnt health-related behaviours.

According to Rosenstock (1974), for somebody to make a health decision, he must first believe that he is susceptible to that particular disease and also that the level of susceptibility is either severe or mild. This particular position was supported by Jegede (1999) when he analyzed three levels of susceptibility. These are:

1) high susceptibility – this is when a person expresses the feeling that he is in real danger of contracting a disease;

2) medium susceptibility – that is a situation when a person believes that even though he is immuned to a disease, yet at a particular moment, he is likely to be adversely tormented; and

3) low susceptibility – this happens when an individual completely denies any possibility of his contracting a disease.

Analysis from this study suggests that certain beliefs especially associated with disease and death have strong effect on maternal and child health. These factors include the conception of MCH; beliefs associated with MCH and certain customs which are harmful to MCH. Among the non-formal educated people, the belief that death is predetermined and that it is beyond human control plays a factor in taking preventive measures against health problems. In the rural communities of Osun State, the people hold the belief that even if a child dies at a tender age and such death is caused, for example, by cholera or any other noticeable illness, it is the destiny, believing that even if the victim had being taken to a standard hospital, he would still die.

Taking therapy is regarded as a mere trial – *ìyànjú lásán*. The action which an individual takes depends on the perceived effect and consequences of such disease. Since the cosmology of disease and illness among the Yoruba does not believe that mortality can occur, due to human health behavior, rather death is predetermined. Hence, many reasons are devised when death occurs. Such include the possession of *Abiku* spirit for children, and *Emèrè* or *Àjé* – witchcraft for maternal death. All these play important factors in taking particular actions concerning the effects and consequences of a particular disease.

Some diseases are regarded as mild and normal, even when symptoms of these diseases which are regarded as mild are the same as serious one. Since there is no scientific proof to distinguish such cases, they are treated with levity until such might have caused irreparable impairment. For instance, diseases like headache, malnutrition especially shortly after weaning, and kwashiorkor, among others are treated as mild and normal. So, these cases are not usually taken to hospital for caring, rather they are referred to traditional medicine or keeping the patients at home using home medication.

Although HBM relates with group attitudes to health care system, yet as HBM explains how and why people take particular therapy but certainly at user's perception of disease, belief system and therapeutic choice, in MCH certain variables are connected with desires to take action in MCH problems. As shown in figure 2 below these variables are analyzed to explain why individual perception and behaviours lead to utilization of MCH services.

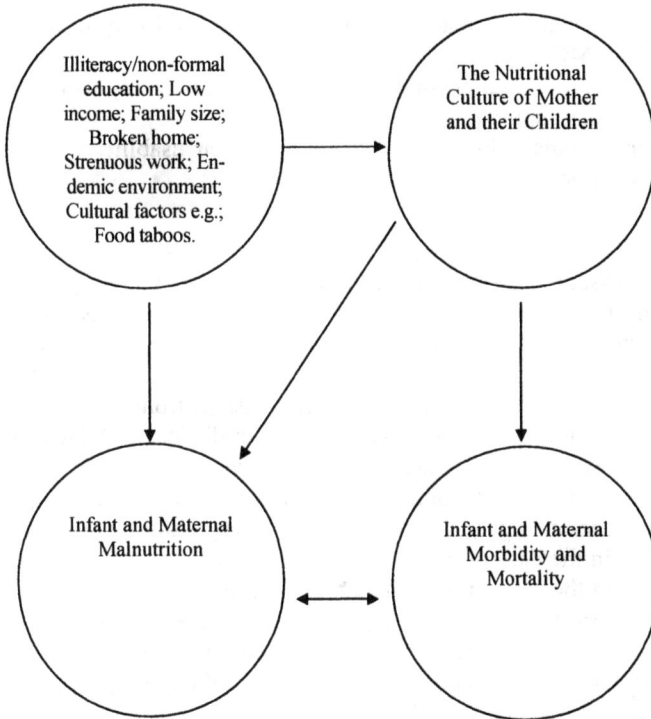

Fig. 2: Social and cultural variables influencing utilization of MCH service

The above conceptual framework explains certain social and cultural variables that are more important to individuals in relationship with group behaviors that causes maternal and child morbidity and mortality. It explains that certain dependent variables such as education, income, family size, occupation and environment may hinder or promote MCH. In actual fact, as indicated in the above model, non-formal education, low income, family size, broken home, food taboos, strenuous work and endemic environment are some dependent variables which determine the nutritional culture of mothers and children. Thus, they lead to infant and maternal malnutrition which may eventually result to infant and maternal morbidity and mortality.

Following the above, the following propositions further explain factors influencing MCH:

1) large family size has greater chance of causing ill-health among the children in that family;
2) income level of the father may affect the health conditions of children and mothers;
3) maternal health information at the household level may have positive effects on MCH system;
4) eradication of common child and maternal diseases may require a multi-disciplinary approach;
5) women's formal education may influence their usability of MCH development programmes in the rural community.

Rural as a Concept

While it is often assumed that it is difficult to define rural communities just like many other concepts in social sciences, it is apparent that rurality is discernible. For clarity and not for the sake of social science dilemma of cultural relativity that makes many of its concepts inappropriately definable, rural communities are those communities that are structurally differentiated from urban in a number of factors which include infrastructural presence; distinct population nature (usually homogenous) and dynamics and location and localization of culture (Ajaga 2004). Thus, rural communities can be identified by predominantly informal economic sector largely driven and relied on agricultural activity either in small scale (as in the case of many rural communities in sub-Saharan Africa) or large scale (as in the case of developed countries and some few intermediate countries of the World); adherence to traditional values and beliefs; low level of technology and infrastructures; widespread poverty (as experience in sub-Saharan Africa); and a small population of less than a thousand people depending on the country's population trends.

The dichotomy between rural and urban communities is therefore clearly marked by the presence of certain facilities meant to improve the quality of life. It is necessary to point out here that there may not be any community where its entire people are equally accessible to high quality of life. However, there is a sharp division in term of access to high quality of life among the people of a particular society based on division marking access to infrastructure. Hence, community that has less quality of life and differentiated by what obtains in another community that has a high quality of life with attendant quantity of infrastructure is thus referred to as rural community. In other words rural communities lack basic needs that sustain healthy living. Economic growth is low while the degree of modernization is equally very slow especially in sub-Saharan Africa. Many of these communities are resilient to changes. Thus, in the word of Ajaga (2004) rural communities are the dens of poverty. In other words rural communities are bedeviled with poverty, where it is assumed that 75% of its population is in dreadful poverty lacking in all basic needs of life such as good health care, shelter, clothing and political power as in the case of Nigeria (Mabogunje 2003).

Following from the above background, the concept of rural, as used in this text refers to the communities in Osun state that fall within the context of the above description. Thus, as stated above, how such rural communities in Osun state manage their health care and their understanding of health in relation to maternal and child health is the central thrust of this text.

2

Research Methodology and Design

Methodology

This work is a descriptive analysis of maternal and child healthcare system among the rural communities of Osun State, Nigeria. It employs qualitative approach with greater emphasis on the use of ethnography. The study employs the community as its unit of analysis. This is as a result of holistic perception of the problem under study. Maternal and child healthcare to a large extent is affected by both etic and emic perceptions associated with healthcare system in the community as a whole, rather than individual or household. Therefore, the aggregate behaviours, attitudes and beliefs associated with the MCH in the study area form the basis of the data. The study covers the period between 1980 and 2008 A.D phased into three stages. 1980-1990 is the first stage, being the period prior the introduction of Primary Health Care (PHC); followed by 1991-2000 the period of active promotion of PHC and 2001-2008, the period when Nigeria entered into another democratic regime with decline in the promotion of PHC programmes and policies.

The combination of emic and etic perspectives enriched the depth of the data, as the perspectives allow the study to examine the conception and practice of healthcare beyond the individual's immediate culture. A greater influence on healthcare system comes from outside. As a result of this assumption, approach focuses on both insiders and outsiders view on equal proportion.

The Study Population

Study population is made up of five categories of respondents namely:
1) Nursing mothers;
2) Health workers both traditional and western;
3) Fathers;
4) Aged men and women;
5) Children between age zero and five.

The principal reason for this categorization was to examine the practice of maternal and child healthcare in historical perspectives. Also to blend both etic perspectives-outsiders' view and emic perspectives-insiders' views of the research subject matter as provided by the inclusion of western and traditional health workers. Children between age zero and five were assessed to corroborate their nutritional status in reference to what their parents asserted.

Rationale for the Choice of the Study Site

Rural communities in Osun state, as the study site, were chosen for three main reasons. Firstly, each of the sites represents each of the administrative zones in Osun State. Secondly, they are rural areas where there exist shortfall of infrastructures and social welfare institutions to support healthcare programmes. They also retain at a greater depth, the practice of traditional culture. Incidentally, each of these sites falls within six local governments selected in 1985 for pilot operation of Primary Health Care (PHC) in Osun State. Therefore, their selections afforded the study an opportunity to assess the performance of PHC.

Osun State has also enjoyed social welfarist policy on health and education being one of the States controlled by Unity Party of Nigeria (UPN) when it was a part of the former Oyo State between 1979 and 1983. The party between 1979 and 1983 introduced free healthcare services in the State. Following this was the establishment of health facilities such as hospitals and many schools. Also, between 1999 and 2003, the then Government of Osun State under the 4th Republic re-established free healthcare with focus on maternal and child healthcare. Therefore, the choice of this research area is to assess how the above changes have affected the development of maternal and child healthcare status especially in the rural communities of Osun state.

Pretest

At the proposing stage of this research, an ethnographic pretest was conducted in the study site. This pilot study involved location of some rural communities in Osun State. During the pilot study, visitation was made to National Population Commission Office; Osogbo where the list of communities identified as rural areas in the State was collected. The study, then selected six communities out of 157 communities identified as rural areas by National Population Commission. The selected communities spread over all the six administrative zones of Osun State. The selection was based on simple random sampling.

Visit to the selected communities showed that only four are typically rural. These are Okinni, Ekusa, Ajaba and Tonkere. Others in the actual sense may not be aptly described as rural, yet they cannot be totally referred to as urban. In this category, a choice of Ibodi and Telemu was made. Those typically rural have poor infrastructures, pure peasant economy, live in traditional lifestyle and depend on the near urban communities such as Ila-Orangun, Inisha, Ilobu and Osogbo among others for livelihood materials. Other communities have some infrastructures such as maternity centers, secondary schools and electricity, but the economy is still peasantry. They also suffer population drift to the nearer urban centers. Some livelihood materials are also sourced from the nearer urban communities. All the above indications then become the rural community identification model. Having noted this problem, the study redesigned the model of community selection. This time, apart from using the administrative zoning in the State, language variation was added.

During the pilot study, examination of child malnutrition was conducted through the available clinical data available in the hospitals. The data confirmed infant mortality though not in conformity with literature-quoted rate. Notwithstanding, casual investigation at this time confirmed the incidence of infant mortality. It was also noted that there was low utilization of healthcare facilities.

To localize the research instruments with the research population, there was a pretest in three research sites. This enabled the study to ascertain the validity and reliability of interview guides. At this level, measurement of response rate was done and questions were re-adapted, to avoid misinterpretations by respondents. The study also restructured the interview guides in order of sequence and priority.

Sampling Procedures

The research involved multi-stage simple random sampling. In the first stage of the random sampling, the selection of the Local Government Areas (LGAs) was made. The second stage involved selection of the communities for the research. The third stage featured the selection of households with the last stage of selection featuring the sampling of research elements. These were done in two categories. The first category was for structured interviews while the second category was the selection of respondents for observational study and unstructured interviews. Household unit is a homestead. In all the six communities, there were 9115 households (PHC 2000) where 300 households were selected for unstructured interview. Another 480 households were randomly selected for household structured interviews.

The sample size was 480 respondents for household structured interview. This was considered adequate for two reasons. It represents one nursing mother out of every five house unit in the research site. This implies that the selection of respondents for structured interview was based on one-fifth-sample frame. The sample frame affords the research a wide coverage with equal chance of selection without overlapping.

Methods of Data Collection

Three main methods of data collection were employed. These were key informants interview, structured interview and observational technique.

Pattern of data collection started with identification of some key informants who served as resource persons through which the study was introduced to the sites. These include the community leaders and identified elites in all the sites. From these resource persons, the study snowballed more key-informants especially the traditional healers, aged women and men, western health workers and some fathers.

Following the key-informants' interview, the research progressed to observational methods through unstructured interviews. During this session, the researcher interacted with 180 nursing mothers sampled from all the research sites.

The last round of data collection strategy was structured interviews with the use of sets of questions formatted into questionnaires. Three hundred respondents were involved in this session.

The three methods complemented each other and helped to ascertain the reliability of data collected typical of triangulation. In the study while key-informant interview generated information regarding specific opinions on individuals, the observational technique particularly worked to generate information on covert attitude through logical deduction of the researcher. The structured interview serves the purpose of documenting the respondents' opinion, which were use to establish tables and illustrations.

Key-Informant Interview

This work relied mostly on key-informant interview to generate information related to the following aspects of the research. Firstly, the use of key informant interview generated information on the local practice of traditional methods of maternal and child healthcare. Secondly, it also generated descriptive data on the practice of MCH in the past and specifically the indigenous knowledge of MCH. Also key-informants were used to generate information on the attitude and practice of western medicine, and the influence of patriarchy on maternal and child healthcare.

The informants were selected purposively and unsystematically simply because the central thrust of the research has no spatial restriction. The sampling was strengthened by snowball approach. Most of the selected informants were those knowledgeable about different aspects of the study.

During the key-informant interview, the study established close social contact with the informants. On the whole, 21 traditional healers, 27 aged women and 32 men (fathers and aged men) and 7 western health workers were involved.

Observational Technique

Being an ethnographic study, I totally immersed myself with the lives of the people within seven months of the fieldwork through observation of their attitudes, knowledge and practices related to maternal and child healthcare. Indeed, I need not to learn the people's language any longer, since I myself speak the same language with the population. Anyway, I only had to readapt my language to the linguistic structures of the people. It was first discovered during the pilot and pretest that my adulterated Yoruba mixed with slang and some English words may affect my data collection. Thus subjected to daily routines of interacting with the study site involving visitations to many hospitals, schools, canteen, beer parlors, and many other places, it becomes possible for the researcher to adapt his language to the local contents and desires.

However, observational technique which was adopted was rather limited. It was not principally participant observation, but rather it was non-participatory observation. Two reasons accounted for this. Firstly, the practices of child and maternal care are not participatory. Secondly, the use of triangulation provided the study with a good opportunity of sourcing for covert attitudes of the people, which was attained through key-informant and structured interviews.

My observational techniques provided the study with opportunity of getting insights and clues for developing questions for structured interview. Similarly, it created the chance of checking and monitoring field information, which became important for evaluation of the collected data.

Since ethnography requires much more than casual observation, the study found out in a great deal more about specific events than could have just been obtained in either key-informant or structured interview. In the process, putting the study propositions in mind in conjunction with the study objectives, I was able to fashion out specific questions concerned with the relationship of events such as the size of family and the frequency of infant morbidity; the level of awareness and utilization of healthcare institution, as well as the beliefs guiding the utilization of a particular healthcare system. In the research site, a total of 180 respondents were specifically observed.

I created elements of representativeness and objectivity in observation by structuring my observations and systematically exploring relationships among different events. These were made possible through meticulous eye-witnessing and interviewing the respondents. I did not rely on my personal memory for recording the site events. I supported my memory with photograph of every important event as well as note-taking of some other crucial events.

Structured Interview

To give the data some degrees of quantification, representativeness and specificity, I involved the use of structured interview in data collection techniques. The interview was based on sampling of one household out of every eight households in the universe where one respondent is selected. Specifically, general questions which generate general responses were asked from the respondents. The target population here was the nursing mothers to elicit more information on their general attitudes related to MCH. This sampling system produced three hundred respondents for interview. Structured interview was conducted after the observation. There were sets of guided questions which were followed. These questions have been tested during the pretest. More general questions came out from observation.

Through structured interview, key-informant data were crosschecked. Responses generated key informants interview were further developed into household interview schedules. Three hundred households were randomly selected from the six communities in the research site based on one-fifth sample frame.

Three interviewers who were University postgraduates assisted in the administration of questions. They were trained for four days prior the days of field research and were involved in the pilot study. The field assistants were relatively knowledgeable in anthropology field investigation. They were young scholars in Anthropology and Sociology Department of Obafemi Awolowo University, Ile-Ife. This is to improve their abilities and skill before the actual fieldwork. They were previously involved in ethnographic studies.

Questions for this household interview elicited information on respondents' personal knowledge, attitudes and practices related to maternal and child healthcare. Questions on socio-economic background of the respondent, therapeutic preference and the use of MCH development programmes were also asked. The most senior wives being the most experienced in each of the polygynous households were selected for interview. Questions were used as corroboration to qualitative data and to generate more general data for easy categorization of our respondents.

Data management and Analysis

All data collected were stored in notebooks and scrutinized before storage into a computer. The Research Assistants were monitored on the field while data collected were checked on daily basis. All collected data were kept strictly confidential. To protect the confidentiality of the respondents, codes were used for questionnaire and interview sheets. Only the Investigators had access to the complete data set that contained the names of respondents. Confidential information relating to their health status and medical records were not released to anyone except members of the research group or those professionals who were providing them essential medical care. No information from the study was communicated or discussed with any spouse or partner of the respondents. For proper handling of qualitative data, all tapes were reviewed at the end of each session to ensure that the recording was good. Notes taken were also reviewed by going through some of the questions randomly with the respondents or participants after every interview to ensure that correct responses were recorded. Each review exercise lasted for about five minutes. All tapes were transcribed verbatim. To check for validity of transcription, 5% of the tapes were re-transcribed by another person to ascertain that the information recorded is accurate.

Data collected were transcribed from tapes and entered into computer using the word pad software before transferring them into text. Responses were tagged and coded subject to similarities. After coding, data were analyzed using the open code software. The research assistants who collected the data from the field and other members of the research group participated in the discussion of the data before the analysis and report writing.

Ethnographic information about the study area

Socio-linguistic Features

The inhabitants of Osun State are predominantly Yorubas. According to the Yoruba myth of creation, it was in this State life begun, credited to Ile-Ife in the earliest beginning. The composition of the population is not different from other Yoruba communities with Yorubas being the largest group of people, where a mixture of other ethnic groups makes up a substantial minority. Other ethnic groups include Igbos, Hausas and Ghanaians among others. Significantly, there are many Fulani settlements found in different locations in the State. These settlements usually have between 10 and 25 people in each of the bands. The bands have close contact and relate with one another.

Osun State as a political unit of Nigerian federation was excised from the old Oyo State in 1991, which was also the break-up of Old Western Region. The Western region before the break-up was composed of Oyo, Egba, Ijebu, Ondo, Ilaje, Ikale, Ekiti, Igbomina and Ife-Ijesa people among other Yoruba sub-ethnic groups. There is little or no cultural variation among these people except the dialect differences, which feature different tonations but similar meanings. Following the creation of Osun state in August 1991, the state is composed of four main Yoruba dialect groups. They are Igbominas spread across the Northern part of the state while the Ife and Ijeshas occupy the South-eastern portion of the state. The fourth group is the Oyo-Yoruba found within the central and western parts of the State.

Osun state is bounded in the North by Kwara State, while the Western border is occupied by Oyo state. In the Southern border, there is Ogun State with Ondo and Ekiti States inhabiting the Eastern border of the state. Like many other Yoruba communities, the Osun people also trace their descendant to the Yoruba progenitor – Oduduwa who was credited with the establishment of Ile-Ife as the cradle of Yoruba civilization. Facial tribal mark is common especially among the elderly people in Osun state. The practice is however fast diminishing among the younger generation. The facial tribal mark features similarities which depict similar traces of lineage. Their facial tribal marks are similar to that of other Yorubas. For instance, the predominant facial tribal marks feature four or three horizontal strokes; four or three longitudinal strokes or four horizontal strokes; and four bars with two-third vertical strokes resting on the topmost horizontal ones. The people are mostly dark in complexion. They have coiled hair, broad nose and moderate head. Their heights range between 5ft and 6ft on the average.

Their dress is a typical Yoruba traditional attire of flowing garments – *Agbádá* with an underwear called *Dansiki* or *Bùbá* worn over *Sòkòtò* (the local pairs of trousers) with *Fìlà* (cap) to match. Occasionally, common among the elders is the use of walking stick called *Òpá*. The local chief (males and females) wears necklaces made of beads as regalia of office – *Àkún*. Women on the other hand dress in wrapper called *Ìró* with headgear *Gèlè* to match and a broad cloth usually placed around the shoulder; this is referred to as *Ìborùn*. Although many young people tend to wear different types of dressing, yet, traditional dresses still remain the most valuable in the society especially for important occasions like marriage, naming and funeral ceremonies. Children use similar attires which are tailored to their sizes.

The people speak four major dialects of Yoruba language. These are Oyo-Yoruba typical of central and western parts of the state. There is also the Ife-Yoruba dialect which is limited to Ile-Ife jurisdiction in the South-eastern part. Ijesha dialect is also located at the extreme Eastern part. The Igbomina Yoruba is the fourth dialect which is located in the Northern axis of the state. In all these dialects, many words are similar in meanings and pronunciations but tonnations differ greatly.

Osun state occupies the western forestry region of Nigeria, providing opportunity for the growth of arable and cash crops. The common arable crops include yams, maize, cassava, plantain, cocoyam, and beans among others. They are made into various staple foods such as pounded yam (*Iyan*), pap (*Eko*); yam or cassava flour (*Elubo*) for *amala;* and beans for (*moinmoin*) or (*akara*) beans cake. The environment similarly provides opportunity for the growth of vegetables such as okra, pepper, tomatoes, *ewedu*, and many species of leafy vegetables. From all these staple foods, *iyan, eba, amala, fufu* and *eko* (both in solid and liquid forms) are the common foods especially in the traditional family setting. These common foods are taken with desired soup to match. Sometimes among this stock of Yoruba, their protein is derived from the bush-meat occasionally trapped or hunted in the bush. To meet the regular supply of bush meat, they usually engage in group hunting.

Their ways of life in terms of attitudes and behaviors have significant influence on their health. For example, accessibility to food in terms of requirements for labor in the farm influences the family sizes, which in turn influences fertility and number of people in the household. Similarly, the mode of dressing protects them against excessive cold which the people usually experience annually between the months of December and February, though subject to seasonal variation. The abundant fauna and flora in their location also provides sufficient herbs for therapy with arable crops making for balanced diet.

Residential Unit

The residential units are compounds, completely demarcated from one another in contiguous manners. A cluster of compounds forms the compound. Each compound is capable of accommodating between one and ten families. Housing within the areas varies but it is typically constructed of mud and bricks, roofed with corrugated iron sheets. Each compound is inhabited by extended family, which have patrilineal relations. The eldest male acts as the head *Báálé*. As a result of modern political system *Báálé* have lost some of their roles especially in criminal adjudications. Some compounds may clutch together to form a quarter which have being changed to political wards represented by a councilor. Although the councilors lack traditional functions in the administration of such quarter, they are nonetheless the representatives of their people in the local council. In some places especially in Telemu, Tonkere and Ibodi, there are chiefs known as *Magaaji* who head the quarters.

The emergence of modern towns has made Osun State to have more towns as urban communities than villages. Two or more of these towns form a local council, except in some towns where municipal councils are found. Typical of such municipal councils are in Ife, Ilesha, Ila-Orangujn, Osogbo, Iwo, Ikirun, Ede, Ilobu and Ejigbo among others. Generally in the State, the traditional rural communities are fast diminishing. They are replaced with modern rural communities where some modern infrastructures are present. These structures are nonetheless inadequate to cater for their people.

Political Organization

The state is made up of autonomous communities numbering thirty which are created into Local Government Councils. Each local government council has a chairman who represents his local government at the State. The State has a Governor based in Osogbo being the capital of the State. Osun state is also zoned into three senatorial districts for the purpose of equitable distributions of development programmes within the state and for selecting a senator from each district to represent the state in the federation of Nigeria. There are also State constituencies at least one from each local government, where a representative is chosen to represent each local government in making law for the State. Each local government is made up of no fewer than eleven wards from where councilors were elected in the administration of their local councils.

Other than the above, there still exist low level of traditional political system practiced in each town and village to compliment the modern political system. In towns, there is a king (*Oba*) being the head of the town while in the village there is *Báálè* also as the head of the village. A chief is selected from each quarter of the town, who forms the council of chiefs. These chiefs together with the head see to the administration of their domains.

Traditional roles accredited to the head include mobilizing his people for community development and passing information to the people. He also arbitrates in small judicial matters which might have not attracted modern litigation. He defends the community land and can alienate such to any individual for residence and farming. The head of a Yoruba community is held in exalted position, which enjoys his people's obedience.

Economic Activities

The people are largely farmers. Their major crops include cash crops like cocoa, oil-palm, cola nut, citrus and plantain, which are still very common in dissident forestry portions of the South, Eastern and Western parts of the State. In other part, the State has witnessed an encroached savannah where food crops such as yams, maize, millet, pepper and tomatoes thrive better. Farmers are found in both towns and villages. The town farmers go to villages where their farms are located in the morning, only to return to the towns in the evening. Village farmers on the other hand stay permanently in the village only to go to town occasionally on Fridays, Saturdays and during any other festivals.

Besides farming, there are also a good number of professional artists and craftsmen, who engage in pottery, basket weaving, palm-wine tapping and many other modern artisanship. Some farmers combine this artisanship with farming in towns. There are also a good number of government workers while such categories are only teachers and health workers in some villages. The commonest feature in the State is the concentration of traditional healers in towns and villages. Only in some towns like Osogbo, Ile-Ife, Iwo, Ede, Ejigbo, Ilesha, Ikirun, there are concentrations of modern hospitals and health clinics.

The average income of the majority of the people was ₦4, 000.00 per annum (FOS 1998) which is ridiculously low especially in the villages. In the town, the average income level is a bit higher than that of the villages. Incomes are generated from the sales of farm produce, petty trading and handicrafts. However, the low level of income does not deter the practice of polygyny. Many people of Osun State expended large sum of their incomes on education of their children before 1999 when the State government declared free education. Free education programme was initially introduced in the state under Awolowo's government in 1955, and in 1979.

Women are subordinate to their husbands; they do not possess economic independence. They lack access to land and they themselves in traditional family setting are sources of labour in their husbands' farms. They usually engage in frying of *Garri*, cracking of palm-nut, palm oil processing, traditional soap making and retailing farm products especially in the villages. In the towns, there are sizeable numbers of women who engage in office work and in big-time retailing. Women however have control on their income. They in fact do not usually turn their income to their husbands. Even when family health is threatened, they always wait for the husband to release money. Only very few, especially those in nuclear and polygynous family use parts of their incomes to assist their husbands especially in family health and in their children's schooling. Husbands make decision for the family regardless of the economic prosperity of a woman. Women regard and submit to the authority of their husbands.

Each of the towns has traditional markets where goods and services are traded. Marketing activities feature people from far distance especially from neighboring States to buy and sell. However, as a result of emergency of new towns as in the case of Osogbo and Ikirun among others, there are changes in market operation. The new towns have shopping centers littered around them. Besides buying and selling in the markets, they are also information centers where basic health information is passed to the people.

Belief System

Just like any other contemporary Yoruba societies, the people have diverse belief systems and religious forms which are shaped by variables like occupation, education and family background. They believe in the Supreme Being known as *Olodumare*. They strongly believe in prayers, invocation, sacrifices, witchcraft and sorcery which are regarded as power with vital forces, which mostly shape people's health and fortunes. They believe that all these powers can invoke illness and bad health on people. The people similarly believe in magic which can be used to promote good or evil and to help and cure. Religious differences fall between Islam, Christianity and Traditional religions. Beliefs associated with these religions have effects on the health seeking behaviours as reported in our findings.

Family

The people are mostly patrilineal. The society features male dominance and mostly male leadership. In this patrilineal society, women lack right to inheritance. Husband is usually regarded as the head of the family. He takes care of his wife or wives and the children. He is the decision-maker for the family with little or no objection from the wife/wives.

Polygynous marriage is commonly practiced among the people. Upon marriage, the right of uxorem and genetricem are absolutely conferred to the husband who might have fulfilled all marriage regulations. This legitimizes the husband's access to sex from his wife without any objection and as such, the husband should claim the fathership of the children raised from such intercourse. Family size in terms of the number of married wife and children are indications of social status for the husbands. As a result of the spread of western education, Christianity and poor state of economy, monogamous marriage is also on the increase. Marriage is usually intra-ethnic especially among the traditional people who marry within their towns or villages. There are modern cases of inter-ethnic marriage, which feature marriage contracted with other ethnic groups.

Among these people, marriage is relatively stable. Although in some cases divorce is allowed. In this case, either of the couples could initiate divorce suit on the grounds of infertility, maltreatment and lost of adequate care among others. Customary courts are vested with determination of marriage suits. The courts can award damages against the husband in most cases.

Selection of Research Sites

The study area was Osun State where six rural communities were randomly selected as the research/study sites. The study sites selected were:
   1) Okinni in Egbedore Local Government in Osun Central zone. Okinni is an Oyo dialect.
   2) Ekusa in Odo-Otin Local Government in Osun Northern zone. The community belongs to Igbomina dialect.
   3) Ajaba which is in Ila Local Government Area, also in Osun Northern zone, in Igbomina dialect of the State.
   4) Tonkere in Ife dialect group of Osun Southern zone in Ayedaade Local Government.
   5) Telemu in Oyo dialect group of Osun Western zone is in Ola-Oluwa Local Government Area.
   6) Ibodi in Ijesha dialect in the Eastern zone of the State. Ibodi is in Atakumosa West Local Government Area.

The selection of the study sites was purposively done to have representation of each of the Yoruba dialectic groups in Osun State. Secondly, the sites have some features of rural settlement. These include low level of infrastructural facilities, predominance of peasant farming and low level of educational resources. These communities as part of their rural nature still suffer rural-urban drift. Similarly, their inhabitants depend on the nearby urban centers to source for their livelihood materials. Significantly, it is noted that all these six communities do not have the same degree of rurality. None of these communities also fall within the scope of traditional rural communities, they are modern rural communities. They are classified as modern rural communities due to the presence of few modern infrastructures. For instance all the communities have primary schools, maternity centers and clinics. Some even have electricity. All these notwithstanding, the predominance of peasant farming, low population density and low level of education of the residents are constant features of their rurality. In Tonkere and Ibodi which are very close to urban settings, the effects are noticed. For instance in Tonkere which is very close to Ile-Ife and particularly close to Obafemi Awolowo University, the frequent movement of people from the community to Ife is a common feature. This ideally has effect on the people's living patterns and access to health care service. Similar situation is present in Ibodi, which is very close to Ilesha. Specifically, the choice of Tonkere and Ibodi as parts of the study sites is principally because they have certain degrees of development ahead of other communities, which are typical and strictly characteristics of modern rural communities. Therefore, they (Tonkere and Ibodi) serve as control test among other categories of rural community. Importantly, the selection of these two sites affords us the opportunity of assessing the utilization of health facilities from the neighboring urban communities.

The third reason for selecting these sites is that each of them fall within each of six administrative zones in the State. And two communities each fall within each of the three senatorial districts in the State. This rationale provides opportunity to examine the political influence on the location of health facilities. Related to the above is the selection of three of these sites as the pioneer sites for Primary Health Care programme in 1985. These are Okinni, Ibodi and Telemu. Two other communities (Tonkere and Ekusa) later have PHC centers since 1998. Ajaba does not have PHC center at all. These features significantly provided opportunities to assess the differential impacts on PHC especially on maternal and child healthcare in the rural communities of Osun state.

The ethnographic information supplied above reveals the social and cultural context of the research site. Certain variables have been explained. Such include belief systems, customs and habits, poverty, education, women social roles and family size. All of these are common denominators found in the research sites, which have effects on maternal and child healthcare in rural communities of Osun State.

The above discussions on the ethnographic information is very essential to the understanding of maternal and child healthcare system in the State. Certain significant socio-cultural variables are noted to have influence on the utilization of maternal and child healthcare services. For instance, the conception of MCH is influenced by belief system, while social and patrilineal structures of the society explain the health decision-making process. The economic system also helps to establish the standard of living of the people and their ability to cope with their health costs.

Ethnography of the Research Sites

Ajaba

Ajaba is in Ila Local Government of Osun State, Nigeria. This community is located in the mid-thick forest part of Eastern axis of the Local Government. It occupies an area of ¼ of a kilometer square at about 14th kilometer distance from Ila-Orangun on the road linking Ila-Orangun and Esa-Oke in Osun State. The people are mainly of the Igbomina sub-Yoruba group in the Northern part of Osun State.

Ajaba derived its name from a river which flows in the community. The original name of the settlement is Kajola. The community was said to have been established in 1963 as a market place by the groups of people from Ila-Orangun, Iresi, Imesi, Koro, Ijero, Igbajo and Otan who decided to establish a village market which will be central to all the communities mentioned above. This decision made the original settlers to name the place *Kajola*, which can be translated to mean "joint wealth".

Having established the market, the people started settling in the community originally as a transit camp, usually a day prior the market day. After the market, they would go back to their different towns. As time went on, people then began permanent residence in Ajaba community. The first person to move to the place and stayed there permanently became the first Baale of Kajola, titled Oloja of Ajaba.

According to 1999 population, Ajaba is occupied by 3,750 people. There are at present many other peoples other than the original settlers in Ajaba. These other peoples include the Igbos, Ghanaians, Tivs and Igala. While Ghanaians and Ibos combined palm wine tapping with farming, Tivs and Igala engaged in hired-labouring.

Political Organization

Ajaba is headed by Oloja of Ajaba who combines the political role with religious functions. He has authority on the people of Ajaba. The Oloja is selected among the Ila-Orangun people in Ajaba. Usually, the eldest among the Ila people becomes Oloja. As at the time of this research, the reigning Oloja was the first appointed Oloja since the community was established. He was appointed in 1964. The community is divided into seven quarters, each quarter belonging to each of the original settlers. Therefore, there is Ila-orangun quarter, Imesi quarter, Iresi quarter, Koro quarter, Ijero quarter, Igbajo quarter and Otan quarter.

Oloja proposes the appointment of village heads that are under him to the Orangun of Ila, who will either confirm or reject the appointment. The Orangun of Ila is the king of Ila who has power over Ajaba and small villages around Ajaba. These villages include *Atoba, Obanla, Alamota, Alagbede, Elejua, Abafa, Idigbon, Aworo-Okun, Aworo-Alase, Odoode, Olumobi, Odosin, Aja-jagun, Obale, Obajinsan, Oba-Orangun, Ejeunwa, Onifare* and *Atere.*

There is individual ownership of both farmland and residential land. New allotment of land is made to a new person by individual who has land without the involvement of Oloja. Oloja too has his own land which he can allot to anybody he wishes. Oloja also settles disputes especially those involving smaller villages under his domain and such disputes involving two quarters or such that may involve a quarter and another village under the domain of Oloja. In such settlement and other palace affairs, Oloja is assisted by his chiefs who he appointed with the community's approval. Oloja has nine traditional chiefs who bear the following titles:

1) Obalumo
2) Odole
3) Obajinmo
4) Oloojoka

5) Oba-Odo
6) Orisawe
7) Obalofin
8) Balogun
9) Odofin

The chiefs are usually selected among the original settlers. Odofin is the second in command to Oloja. He acts for Oloja when Oloja is out of the community.

Socio-Economic Development

Major occupation in Ajaba is farming for men while women assist their husbands in the farm. Some men engage in buying and selling of cocoa, palm oil and palm kernel. Women also engage in selling of petty items such as beverages, cigarettes and some other household materials. They also engage in the production of palm oil. The chief crops cultivated in Ajaba include cocoa, kolanut, oil-palm, yam, cocoyam, maize, plantain, vegetable and pepper.

In 1963, a local market was established in Ajaba which serves as a meeting point for many people for exchange of goods and services. The market grew up fastly because of availability of farm products. Between 1963 and 1964, an untarred road was constructed between Ila-Orangun passing through Ajaba to Esa-Oke in the then Old Western Region. As at the time of research, this road was still an earth road till present with gullies and potholes.

In 1965, a local primary school was established through communal efforts. The school served Ajaba people and villages under Ajaba. In 1980, a secondary school was established. In 1982, a maternity and dispensary centre was also established while in 1995, a 25-bed Health Centre was awarded for construction. The project is still under construction as at the time of the study.

The community has no pipe borne water or modern borehole. The source of water is Ajaba River which is almost a kilometer away from the centre of the community. The river does not have capacity to flow all year round. The community keeps on locally drilled well when the river dries up.

Cultural Attitudes Related to Health Care

The people of Ajaba are the brand of Yoruba known as Igbomina. They practice polygyny. On the average, a family is composed of 13 people made of a father, two or more wives and 10 children. Marriage is mostly guided by the Yoruba intra-group marital rules and contracted through various regulations and practices. The people are patrilineal which feature male dominance and male leadership. Husband in the household is the head of the household and he is responsible for decision taking especially in healthcare. The family size has influence on household health care financing.

Residential Pattern
Ajaba community was established specifically at a junction. The topography of the land depicts a table-land environment, free of hills, valleys and mountains. Therefore, the settlement pattern shows a circular arrangement with houses clustered together. Some portions of the market place are open and not permanently occupied. Other portions of the community are designated into school area, religious ground, hospital and housing areas.

The school area occupies both the primary and secondary school while religious ground has the Muslim prayer ground on one part and at the other part, there is a church. Hospital area is where dispensary, maternity and health centres were built. The housing area forms the largest space where mostly residential houses for living were built. The housing pattern shows mud wall with majority facing the main road. According to an informant, housing pattern prevents the houses from thunderstorm. The living population concentrated in the centre of the community.

Ekusa
The Ekusa aborigines were from Empe community in Nupe Kingdom of Niger State in Nigeria. There were originally three brothers who fled Empe as a result of incessant child mortality. The three brothers decided to leave Empe southward to the then Oyo Kingdom which was famous then. Historical correlations had been in existence between Nupe and the Yoruba in Old Oyo Empire. The popular correlation is the marital link between Sango, one time Oyo king and Oya, a Nupe woman (Ajala 2001). There are many other Yoruba towns having historical links with Nupe people.

As they were coming, they came through the northern penetration of the Old Oyo Empire and on getting to Ofa in Ibolo province he was made as the *Eesa* – traditional chief of Ofa. The other two proceeded southwards. They came to a place called Igbaye which is about 10 kilometre from the present location of Ekusa. They settled therein and engaged in farming.

One of the two brothers again fled Igbaye to a new and virgin land following the problem of child mortality which he suffered in Igbaye. He eventually settled and built a hut to accommodate him. He was in this place where he farmed and established his family.

Long after he had settled, there was a visit of a dancing masquerade known as *Egun-Oje* to the community for dance performance. But the masquerade was rejected. In annoyance, when the masquerade was going, it invoked the spirit and cursed the community with smallpox. Smallpox then ravaged the community and caused high mortality. The people then decided to leave the place. They eventually dispersed to several places which included Okuku, Ikirun and Inisa. After the ravage subsided, they went back to the community.

On getting back, they met some of their people who did not run away during the crisis. They were surprised and exclaimed *E ku e sa* that is, "you still re-mained here, you did not run away". The remark *E ku e sa* thereby became the name of this community. Following usage over time, the term was assimilated into Ekusa, which is the community's name till today. Ekusa is located in Odo-Otin Local Government Area in the northern part of Osun State. The community has a population of 9,279 people.

Economic Activities

Economy of this community is peasantry. Men and women engage in fragmenta-ry small-scale farming. They produce crops like cocoa, kolanut and leafy vege-tables. Maize, cowpea and millet also grow very well in this community. Men are typically known for cultivation of cash crops, when women engaged in vege-tables. Women similarly engage in black-soap making, palm oil processing and cracking of palm kernel.

Women also engage in petty trading of household needs. There is a local market which is attended every five days. In this market, exchanges of goods are conducted. The market usually attracts traders from Okuku, Inisha, Osogbo and Ikirun; and from other neighbouring villages and towns.

Political Organization

Political organization in Ekusa is not different from that of any other Yoruba town. In the traditional setting, there is king – *Oba* titled Elekusa of Ekusa. The Oba is selected from one of the royal families. Oba is the head of the communi-ty. He sees to the day-to-day administration of the community. He maintains law and order in the community as well as seeing to the development of the town. He also has both religious and judicial roles. He mediates and solves disputes emanating among his subjects.

The king is assisted by kings. In Ekusa, there are two sects of chiefs. The first sect is the kingmakers (*Afobaje*) while the second sect is the regular chiefs who are vested with daily administration of the town. The kingmakers are only vested with selection and crowning of a new king.

Socio-Economic Development

In 1925, a primary school was established in Ekusa, following the increase in population and the yearnings of the people to have western education. Also in 1945, another primary school was established. In 1982, a secondary grammar school was established while in 1991, electricity was extended to Ekusa from Okuku. There is no pipe borne water in Ekusa. The community relies on bore-holes constructed by Directorate of Food, Roads and Rural Infrastructure (DFFRI).

Belief System Associated with Health Care
Ekusa is noted for the practice of separatist churches. Among these are Kerubim
and Seraphim, Aladura churches and Celestial Church of Christ. The people especially mothers and children practice faith-healing. There are also traditional
healers and Elewe-omo who explores the fauna and flora found in this environment into making of herbs and mixtures for various types of ailments. Common
diseases in Ekusa include malaria, typhoid, dysentery, diarrhea, cholera and
chicken pox. There are maternity and dispensary centres in Ekusa.

Ibodi
Ibodi is situated at sixth kilometer from Osu on the road linking Osu with Ilesa.
The community is also about eight kilometer to Ilesa starting from Owa's Palace
in Ilesa township. Ibodi was said to be founded in around 17th century. According to oral tradition, a group of seven men with their wives headed by a man
called Isidale left Ile-Ife in search of virgin farmland. Like others, Isidale was a
farmer and warrior. They moved eastward of Ile-Ife from an Ile-Ife quarter
known as Ilolomu. Among the seven men was an Ifa priest who usually consulted oracle to know the place where they should settle.
      When the group got to the present settlement, they consulted the Ifa priest
who divined if the place was good for habitation. The oracle revealed that the
place was good and that there was another place within a close distance which
was equally good. So, the people had to decide as to whether to stay or move to
the close distance. Some of the people supported settling in the first place while
some others wanted to group to move to the other place. To avoid conflict and
division, Ifa priest then suggested that the people should vote to reach a decision. They obliged to the priest suggestion, so they voted. The winning vote was
in favour of the first place, hence the people called the place *Ibo didi* place,
meaning where we voted to stay. The name upon usage assimilated to what is
presently called *Ibodi*.
      Isidale was made the first king of the community. He gave birth to only one
son named Oloja who succeeded his father and established the kingship lineage
in Ibodi. Since the demise of Isidale, Ibodi has installed almost 50 kings up to
the present.
      Ibodi community was occupied by a population estimated to about 8,270
people. This population includes non-Yoruba such as Ibo, Tiv and Igala people.
Ibodi people are the Ife-Ijesa brand of Yoruba whose linguistic dialect is not the
same as that of Igbominas.

Socio-Economic Development
The principal occupation in Ibodi is farming. Both men and women are involved
in farming. Men are engaged in both cash and food cropping. Women do not
have right to cultivate cash crop. They only engage in food cropping. Chief

among the cash crops being cultivated include cocoa, oil palm, kolanut, cashew and plantain. Common food crops include yam, cocoyam, maize, cassava, vegetable, tomatoes and pepper. Women also engage in petty trading and cloth weaving, while men mostly engage in buying and selling of cocoa. There is a local market for the community where exchanges of goods are transacted.

In 1920, the road that runs through the community from Ile-Ife to Ilesa was constructed while in 1927, a primary school was established. In 1980, there was an extension of electricity from Ilesa to Ibodi and in 1981, a dispensary and maternity centre was established in Ibodi.

Political Organization
Ibodi is a major village which has many other villages under its control. These villages include *Ilofin, Imuro, Ile-oke, Isua, Oke-aku, Idila, Oloyin, Olorombo* and Imusan. The Oloja of Ibodi is held responsible for the affairs of these villages. He reports to Owa Obokun of Ijeshaland in Ilesha.

Ibodi is headed by Oloja of Ibodi who is assisted by compound heads. There were 15 compound heads heading each of the 15 compounds in Ibodi. Each compound is made up of patrilineage people numbering between fourteen and thirty-two members. There are other members who are not of the same patrilineage in a compound. These other people are usually non-natives of Ibodi.

Oloja of Ibodi functions as political, religious and social leader. He represents his community at the Local Government and in Owa's palace in Ilesha. He has control over the land, although not absolute control. He settles disputes involving individuals and that involving smaller villages under his jurisdiction.

Residential Pattern
The community is arranged in lineal form. Houses scattered both left and right sides of Ibodi/Ilesa road that runs through the community. Farmland is far from residential area. Houses are built of mud bricks made of red clay and roofed with corrugated iron sheets.

Okinni
The people of Okinni came from Oyo Alaafin during the reign of Ajaka, onetime king of Oyo Kingdom. There were only three people headed by a farmer and hunter called *Orunmoyeniyi*, who first settled in Okinni. Orunmoyeniyi led the people to the present site of Okinni.

Orunmoyeniyi left Oyo because he was affected by child mortality which was linked to *Abiku*. He consulted Ifa oracle who told him to leave Oyo if he wanted to have children. Ifa further directed him to move westward of Oyo, to a place where he would found peacock. There he should settle and establish. In his attempt to comply with the oracle, he solicited for the support of his two friends who agreed to follow him. The three men then took off their journey with their wives until they got to a place where they found a peacock. Yoruba name for peacock is *Okin*, so when they saw *Okin*, they shouted *Okin ni in* meaning "This is peacock". That is where the community derived its name which is assimilated over the time to mean *Okinni*.

Okinni is founded on tableland covered with overgrown trees and shrubs in their original forms. Oral tradition further stated that there were rich fauna in the place at the earliest occupation. However, at present due to farming and other human activities, the community is covered with dissident forest and relatively turning to grassland where there are intensive farming.

Okinni is bounded in the east by Ojutu River which borders Ilobu and Okinni River in the West where the community shares boundary with Woru village. In the North it shares boundary with Oba River, where the community also shares border with Igbokiti village.

The present population of the community stands at 12,520 (NPC 2006) people comprising many other Yoruba groups and non-Yoruba groups.

Okinni town is located at kilometer five from Osogbo on Osogbo-Ilobu Road. It is situated in Egbedore Local Government of Osun State. Predominantly, the people of Okinni speak Yoruba-Oyo dialect.

This people's ways of life are similar with other Oyo Yoruba in Nigeria. The marriage pattern is local exogamy which is mostly polygynous. Marriage ceremony is celebrated with a lot of cultural activities such as nuptial poetry – *Rara sunsun*; the display of traditional dress and many other festive moods. In traditional setting, a woman is expected to keep her virginity until she marries but this tradition has been weakened by the prevalence of adolescent sexuality.

Economic Activities

The people of Okinni are largely farmers who major in tendering both cash and food crops. Their principal cash crops include cocoa, oil-palm, kolanut, citrus and plantain. Food crops include yam, cowpea, maize, sweet potato, pepper and leafy vegetables. Cassava is cultivated extensively. The influence of urban communities surrounding Okinni reflects in other economic activities being practiced in the present-day Okinni. These activities include trading in petty household items and many other artisanship. These urban locations such as Osogbo, Ilobu, Erin and Ede serve as markets for bulk purchasing of these household items.

There is gender distinction in the people's economic activities. In the traditional pattern, women are not engaged in serious and tedious farming activities. They were engaged in what is referred to as simple food cropping such as pepper and leafy vegetables. Women's major function in a traditional household is to assist their husbands in farm work. They are engaged in harvesting and transportation of farm produce from the farms to the village. Also, they help their husbands to sell the products. They also engage in processing of raw foods such as yam-powder and Garri for household consumption and for sales on behalf of their husbands. Women are also engaged in traditional soap making and palm kernel cracking through manual processing. These practices are still prevalent at present. On the other hand, men only cultivate farms.

At present, the community has some institutions such as schools, maternity center, palm-oil processing factory, livestock poultries and local markets.

Political Organization

Okinni is politically organized in Yoruba traditional kingship pattern. The king (*Oba*) heads the community. He has the authority to keep the community in order. Oba is selected from royal family. The community has seven male children from the founder – Orunmoyeniyi, who was the first *Oba* of the community. The selection of a new Oba is done after the demise of the incumbent Oba. His selection is made from adult males among those in one of the seven royal families. The practice favors rotational system based on the seniority among the royal families and seniority among the surviving males in the royal family where the new Oba is to emerge. The selection of a new Oba is done after consulting Ifa divination that might have approved the suggested name. The Kingmakers are also present to ratify the selection. Kingmakers are made of seven traditional chiefs. These are *Eesa, Jagun, Otun, Ekerin Odofin, Akogun* and *Iyalode*. The Kingmakers (*Afobaje*) also function in traditional chief council.

Oba performs religious, political and social roles in the community. He represents his community in meetings of Obas in the State. He is the symbol of traditions and unity in the community. He is highly respected. He resides in a big compound built and maintained by the community. The compound is called *Aafin*. Aafin is edified with historical monuments to display the rich cultural heritage of the Okinni people. Oba is vested with the duty of dispute settlements arising from individual interactions with others. Such may include matrimonial cause, disputes on property or intra-community feuds. He may also mediate in inter-community crises involving his community and others.

The king owns the land. He is the owner of the land where Okinni has jurisdiction. However, the land is shared among the seven royal families who act in trust on the management of the land allocated to each royal family. Each royal family still assigns the land in its care to segmented families belonging to each of them. The new allotee pays royalty to the King through the family head who manages that particular allotment. Land in Okinni is used for various purposes which include farming, residential and religious functions.

Each compound in Okinni has its head known as *Baale. Baale* is responsible to the King and handles small matters concerning the maintenance of peace and order in the compound unit. Political information is disseminated to the people through the use of town crier who attracts the people's attention with the use of gongs.

Socio-economic Development

Okinni was established in the late 16th century or so. Since then, many socio-economic infrastructures have sprung up. The community has expanded in its size from two original houses to almost 3,712 house units scattered within the community. The housing pattern has changed considerably. In the traditional setting, it was mud-walled, with grass-thatched roof. Houses then were not with ceiling or plastering. Cow dung was used to keep dust from the floor. Many houses were in bungalow shape with very tiny windows called *Marasana*. Presently, most houses are built of concrete cement, roofed with corrugated iron sheets and plastered. Though not many houses were painted even as at the time of research, yet there is a remarkable improvement from the traditional style. As at 2007 there were some bungalow flat buildings with perimeter fencing and more decent with modern outlooks now found in the township.

Road networks have also been improved from a single earth pedestrian jungle which existed in the community in the 16th century till late 18th century. The construction of Osogbo-Ilobu-Ogbomoso road in the early 19th century opened Okinni community to more roads being constructed to link the community with Osogbo/Ilobu-Ogbomoso road, which is ¼ of a kilometer distance to Okinni main town, as the community has spread to the road bypass.

With the upsurge of more people resident in the community, the community now has two primary schools. The first school was built in 1922. Secondary Grammar School was also built in 1981 while churches, dispensary and maternity centers were also established. Electricity was extended to Okinni from Osogbo in 1992. The extension of electricity saw the establishment of cottage agro-allied industries in the community. Such include poultry farms, palm oil mills and bakery.

Health Behaviour and Attitude

Okinni is close to two big Rivers – River Ojutu where the community shares borders with Ilobu, and Oba River which is currently dammed by Osun State Government as Hydro-pressure booster to Ede dam in the State. These two rivers are linked with the prevalence of Onchocerciasis in Okinni. There are also pockets of Fulani settlements with their cattle around this community. This creates recipe for tsetse fly breeding which is capable of transmitting Onchocerciasis.

Despite the closeness of this community to water dam, Okinni still lacks regular flow of pipe-borne water. The water base in the community is low thus creating problem of getting enough water in wells. The community therefore relies on brooks and streams for domestic needs of water. This in the past had caused the outbreak of cholera and similar water-borne diseases. Rheumatism and chickenpox were said to have broken out in Okinni several occasions in the past. The use of dump-hills and nearby bush for excretion further put the community's hygiene in danger.

Telemu

The original settlers of Telemu were said to have migrated from Orile-Owu in the present-day Isokan Local Government of Osun State at the Eastern border of Osun State with Ogun State in Nigeria. Orile-Owu is presently estimated to cover a distance of about fifty kilometer from the present location of Telemu. Oral history has it that at somewhat around 15th century, there was a royal tussle which broke out as a result of vacant stool of Olowu of Orile-Owu which was contested for. The loosing contestants felt that they were cheated, and then they vacated Orile-Owu for an unknown destination. The migrants were led by a hunter known and called *Anlugba Akindele*. *Anlugba Akindele* was a fearless and valiant hunter. On his travelling, he passed through Ode-Omu and Northward towards Iwo town. On the way, Anlugba and his entourage felt tired and stopped at a place to relax. When they regained their strength, they furthered their journey.

After moving for some time, they discovered that Anlugba had left his walking stick where they stopped to relax. So Anlugba sent one of his followers to go and pick the stick. The person sent could not go back alone for fear of wild animals and forest evils, so another person was asked to *Te le mu* that is to follow him and picked it. The name got assimilated and contrasted to be called Telemu till today. Later, due to the power of Anlugba, the name Alefoofoo was added to the name Telemu. Thus, the community became Telemu Alefoofoo.

In 1830, the community was invaded by Fulani Jihadists and the people fled the community for nearby places for refuge. After six years the refugees came back to resettle in the original settlement. This time around, there was an expansion in the community and the traditional heritages of the past were kept. The community then was renamed as Telemu Agbanda. Agbanda was said to have led his people to resettle in Telemu following the first Fulani invasion.

However, ten years after this resettlement, a group of masquerade dancers visited the community to perform but they were refused enterance. In annoyance, the masquerade dancers cursed the community with smallpox and the people having been ravaged had to desert the community again. When the crisis subsided, they came back and the people at that time were led by Olupemo. This third resettlement has since then remained Telemu till today.

Before the destruction of Telemu Alefoofoo, the community had grown so large with almost one hundred and forty blacksmith centres located in the community then. These sites still reflected in Telemu with occasional discovery of material remains related to this technology. To confirm and establish this claim, there is need for archaeological expedition in this community.

The above suggests that Telemu is an ancient town presently occupying an area measuring about three square kilometers to the North-East of Iwo, within a distance of about 55 kilometres distance from Ibadan. It is also lying within 35 kilometres South of Osogbo on Osogbo-Iwo-Ibadan road and 55 kilometres away from Oyo township.

Telemu people are brands of Oyo Yoruba whose dialects have close similarities with other central Yoruba. There exists other cultural relatedness with other central Yoruba. Such include tribal marks of different versions such as four horizontal or four vertical strokes and seven horizontal strokes with cross bars. Patterns of dressing reflect men wearing *agbada, sapara, buba* and *sokoto* with caps to match. Women usually wear *iro* and *buba* and *gele* to match.

Dietary habit of the people is largely detemined by what their ecosystem produces. Therefore, common foods are maize paste, pounded yam, *amala, eba*, cowpea processed into *moin-moin* or *ekuru*. Environment still makes the production of leafy vegetables and varieties of fruit available as micro-nutrient foods.

Political Structure

The political structure of this community is not different from that of other Yoruba communities. There is Oba who is not a beaded-crown Oba. He has both political and religious functions in the community. He also manages the community's joint resources such as land, market and stream. There are traditional chiefs who assist Oba in community administration.

Economic Activities

Telemu is an agrarian community with vast acreage of land for farming. In the past, substantial part of this land was virgin groove with thick and woody plant which entirely formed shade with little or no space for deem of light to reflect on the land surface. The fragments of ritual forests in the community today show the tree climbers of various species enriching the soil fertility in the past.

Due to intensive agricultural activity competition for land resources, competition for land has diminished the traditional forest heritage in favor of dissident forest now showing secondary flora. There are still some woody species of trees and palms which were cultivated to produce cash crops. Such include oil-palm, cocoa, cashew and kolanut. These cash crops are inter-cropped with some food crops which include yam, maize, cassava, cowpea and cocoyam.

The people practice cooperative labor in their farm management. Also, there is a sharp division of labor largely determined by sex and the age of the members of a typical household. For instance, women do not cultivate cash crops but only food crops. Women specifically engage in food processing, reproduction and child tendering. They are also the marketers of their husband's farm produces apart from cocoa.

The practice of slash and burn farming is still prevalent while farm-holding is fragmentary. The system favors constant shift from one farmland which might have been tilled for some years and left for fallowing before returning to such land after four or five years of desertion.

Infrastructural Development

In 1920, a primary school was established followed by another primary school in 1955. In 1977, a public secondary school was also established. In 1998, the community through communal efforts established another Grammar School.

Health care institutions established in the town include St. Zenos Primary Health Center which was established and managed by Catholic Church in the town. The town also has maternity and dispensary centers while another 60-bed hospital is under construction. There is also a private clinic in the town. The community also has pipe-borne water which does not flow regularly. The people rely more on wells and stream water. In 1978, there was an extension of electricity to the town.

Tonkere

Tonkere is situated in the heart of forest in Ayedaade Local Government of Osun State. The community is bounded in the West by Obafemi Awolowo University campus, Ile-Ife, in the East by Ayetoro and in the North by Edunabon. The community has a population of about 7,280 people according to National Population Projection (NPC 2006).

Some villagers, who had earlier occupied different locations such as Akinloye, Oyewole, Igbintayo, Adekemi, Osunade, Joojoo, Keesi and Adesigun villages all in Ife division, established this community in 1928. All these villages are still in existence. These villages came together in 1928 to establish a common market. The site of the market was selected close to a flowing stream known as Tonkere. As time went on, the market saw the settlement of people and eventually becomes a permanent settlement. It was formerly named Oluwatedo, but for the popularity of Tonkere stream, the name Tonkere overshadowed former name and Tonkere becomes the popular name for the community.

The original settlers were from Modakeke town near Ile-Ife in the present-day Osun State. People from many other places have however came to settle in Tonkere. These include Edunabon and Gbongan. Presently, the inhabitants include Ibos and Togolese who engage in palm-wine tapping and hired labour.

Political Organization

Tonkere is headed by a village head titled *Baale*. *Baale* is selected among the oldest compound heads in the community. There are only seven quarters, each headed by *Baale* (compound head). All the compound heads are the palace chiefs to the community head – *Baale*.

Baale performs political, social and religious functions. He sees to the growth of the local market in Tonkere. He settles disputes. He also represents his community in all occasions involving Tonkere and other communities. He enjoys the support of his people and the people treat him with respect and dignity. He is the most honoured in the community. He receives annual tributes from his subjects.

Economic Activities

The forest region where Tonkere is located is more favorable to farming. The people cultivate mainly cash crops such as cocoa, kolanut, plantain, cashew, oil palm and oranges which thrive very well. The use of hired labor is predominant. They also engage in production of food crops such as millet, yam, maize, cassava and leafy vegetables.

Men are saddled with the responsibility of crop cultivation, women practice in harvesting and selling of farm products. Women are also engaged with processing of foods for consumption and for sales.

Infrastructural Development in Tonkere

Following the establishment of a community market in 1928, a primary school named St. James Primary School was established in 1930. In 1935, the road linking Tonkere-Ayetoro and Akoda was constructed through communal efforts while in 1938; another road linking Tonkere with Edunabon was also constructed. The establishment of University of Ife in 1964 which is now Obafemi Awolowo University sited at about seven kilometers to Tonkere made Tonkere people and other villages to construct another road from the University Southgate to Tonkere in 1968. In the same year, a Grammar school was established in the town. Churches were also established. At present, some of the churches include The Apostolic Church, Christ Apostolic Church and The Anglican Church.   In 1980, a dispensary and maternity centre was established while in 1991, the Government of Osun State embarked on the construction of Health Care Centre, the project which has not been completed as at the time of research.

In 2000, Osun State Government commenced the construction of rural housing project in this community. The project was under construction as at the time of research. Earlier in 1998, the United Nations Development Programs (UNDP) built Garri processing industry with modern technical equipment for the processing of cassava to Garri in the town. UNDP also constructed boreholes which now serve the people with water.

Demographic Characteristics of the Respondents

A total of 567 respondents were interviewed. Out of these 567, there were 81 men and 486 women. Seventy-nine percent of the men had no formal educational training while 78.2 percent of the women fall within the same category. Only 21 percent of the men had formal education while only 21.7 percent of the women also had formal educational training. Majority of the men had married (74.1 percent); also 79.8 percent of the women respondents had married. The average percentage of married respondents was 79.0 percent, while 10.0 percent of the total respondents were either divorcee or widows with women divorcee averaging 7.4 percent. Only 12.8 percent (62) female respondents were unmarried.

Only 9.9% (8) male respondents had one wife while 24.7 percent had two wives and 50.6% had three wives with 12.3 percent having four wives and 2.5 percent having five wives. Out of 480 households selected for the interview, 17.6 percent of the households (85) have between one and five children, 186 households (38.8 percent) had between six and ten children per household. The households that had between 11 and 15 children each accounted for 23 percent (110). Only 20.6 percent had between 16 and 20 children each. Rural communities in Osun state were mostly Muslim dominated with an average of 75.3 percent of the respondents being Muslims. Only 14.8 percent were Christians, with only 9.9 percent favoring traditional religion.

The income levels of the male respondents reflect 25.9 percent earning less than ₦1,000.00; while 30.9 percent earned between ₦1,000.00 and ₦2,000.00. Only 18.6 percent of the respondents earned between ₦2,000.00 and ₦3,000.00. With only 10.0 percent earning between ₦3,000.00 – ₦4,000.00 and 8.7 percent of the male respondents earned more than ₦3,000.00 per month. The female respondents had 23.7 percent earning less than ₦1,000.00 with only 27.0 percent earning between ₦1,000.00 and ₦2,000.00, only 20.0% of our female respondents earned between ₦3,000.00 and ₦4,000.00 while 5.3 percent of our female respondents earned more than ₦4,000.00. The incomes imply that 75.3 percent of our male respondents were below poverty level of less than U.S. $30 monthly income (UNICEF 1999) while 74.7 percent of our female respondents fell below the poverty level of US $30 monthly income.

Majority of the respondents practiced farming (69.1 percent for male; 68.3 percent for females) while 11.1 percent of male respondents engaged in trading, with only 18.5 percent of female respondents doing the same. Only 7.4 percent engaged in office work among the male respondents while only 3.1 percent among the female respondents also engaged in office work. Among the men, only 12.3 percent were artisans with 10.1 percent of the women being artisans.

From the socio-demographic characteristics of the respondents, the rural people of Osun State have peculiar features which definitely have effects on their maternal and child healthcare system. 79.0 percent and 78.3 percent men

46   Rural Health Provisioning

and women respectively without formal education, combined with income levels
of 75.3 percent (men) and 74.7 percent (women) below the poverty line. In conjunction with large family size which the income levels could not cope with,
their conceptions of maternal and child health care are greatly affected. These
cultural features also influenced the utilization of maternal and child healthcare
services in rural communities of Osun State.

Table 1: Demographic Characteristics of the Respondents

Variables	Men (N = 81)	(%)	Women (N=486)	%	Total (N=567)	%
AGE						
15-20	8	9.9	85	17.85	93	
21-30	19	23.5	157	32.3	176	27.4
31-40	26	32.1	118	24.3	144	55.8
41-50	12	14.8	58	11.9	70	56.4
51-60	5	6.2	42	8.6	47	26.7
61-70	8	9.9	17	3.4	25	14.8
>70	3	3.7	9	1.8	12	13.3
TOTAL	81		486		567	5.6
WESTERN EDUCATION						
Married	60	74.1	388	78.8	448	79.0
Divorced/ Widow	21	25.9	36	7.4	57	10.0
Unmarried	-	-	62	12.8	62	11.0
WIVES/HOUSEHOLD						
1	8	9.9				
2	20	24.7				
3	41	50.6				
4	10	12.3				
5	27	2.5				
>5	NIL	-				
CHILDREN/HOUSEHOLD						
No. of Children	(480)	17.6				
1-5	85	38.6				
6-10	186	23.0				
11-15	110	20.6				
16-20	99					
OCCUPATION						
Farming	56	69.1	332	68.3	338	68.4
Trading	9	11.14.200	90	18.5	99	17.4
Office Work	6	17.4	15	3.1	21	3.7
Artisans	10	12.3	49	10.1	59	10.4
Christians	12	14.8	72	14.8	84	14.8
Moslems	61	75.3	364	75.1	425	75.1
Traditional	8	9.9	50	10.3	58	10.2

3

Culture and Health

Introduction

To establish background knowledge for the study and the need to enrich knowledge on the subject-matter, an exploration has been made into some existing secondary sources of data. Areas such as medicine and culture, traditional medicine and social change, maternal and child healthcare in Nigeria, MCH development programmes in Nigeria and critiques of the explored texts are covered. Hence this chapter relies on secondary sources of information.

Medicine and Culture

The relevance of behavioral science has been noticed in the development of health care programmes and in the control and prevention of diseases as far back as 50 years ago (More 1967; Otite 1987; Twaddle 1982; Oke 1993, 1996). This position was made possible as a result of the discovery of the association and convergence between medicine and culture which applied anthropologists have intensified in a great deal. Survey of various definitions of culture has confirmed that culture comprises of systems of shared ideals, system of concepts, rules and meanings that underlie and explain human lives (Embers 1978).

Culture is a set of systems, values, principles, rules and all other capabilities which people of a particular setting have come to inherit from their predecessors and through which they have come to illustrate how they live and do what they do, and how they relate with others, other than their immediate individuals. Medicine is an aspect of culture (Embers 1978; Oke 1978; Read 1966). In this way, to understand bio-cultural phenomena such as medicine and disease, one needs to consider cultural pattern specific of an environment (Ajala 2006; Ajala 2007). Jegede (1998) noted that culture of a particular group of people at a specific period of time always influences a particular way of living in that society. He further noted that economy, which is a dynamic phenomenon, is more of an indicating factor of illness and health.

In their explanation of health, Patrick and Wickizer (1995) noted certain elements which influence the health of the people. Cultural elements such as social class, gender inequalities and racism are considered as basic determining elements of health. These are mainly the networks of social relations. House et al (1988) similarly noted that social networks and social support can affect mortality, psychological and physical functioning, health perceptions and how individuals and families management of disease and illness are held.

Still on the convergence between health and culture, the Canadian Government (1974) through analytic framework published as *A New Perspective on the*

Health of Canadians offered a useful means of classifying the major determinants of health using the categories of life style, environment, human biology and healthcare organization. It was this framework which Evans and Stoddart (1990) developed into more detailed model. The causal model provides a sound conceptual basis for considering the influence of culture on health. As a determinant of health, cultural interactions are the broader determinants of health. Notably cultural elements such as occupation, education, family size and host of other social institutions are social influences that affect the health and well-being of individuals. In this respect, Evans and Stoddart (1990) consider individuals, groups and agents as recipients of cultural influence that in turn affect people's health. Culture also incorporates the physical environment in which individual lives are faced with socio-biological infirmities. Hence, health is defined as general conditions of well-being and not mere absence of biological disconformities. Such conditions include physical, social, political and in fact infrastructural.

In view of the relationship between medicine and culture, medicine and illness are viewed from general and holistic perspective. Hence, the redefinition of the concept, health as not only the absence of biological infirmity, but much more generally, the complete state of well-being which include psychological, biological, economic, political and social states of well-being (WHO 1978). It suggests that based on cultural understanding, every society has a specific way of tackling its medical problems. This practice may be indigenous and triable medical practices and/or diffused foreign medical system.

Traditional Medicine and Social Change
Traditional medicine exists with time with enough data abound worldwide to ascertain its efficacy. The Ayurvedic in India, acupuncture in China and *Elewe omo* in Yoruba of Nigeria have been studied and announced to be meeting the health requirement of vast majority of people using them. Utility and potency of native medicine have also been noticed by many authors (Bonsi 1982; Owumi 1993; Oke 1995; Pearce 1986; Odebiyi 1977).

There are differing terminologies by different authorities on traditional medicine. While some refer to it as native medicine, indigenous and primitive medicine, others refer to traditional medicine as folk, black medicine and in extreme cases *juju* (Owumi 1993). Upon this background, the traditional medicine is conceived as sum total of all knowledge and practices whether explicable or not, used in the diagnosis, prevention and management of physical and mental imbalances which are relying exclusively on practical experience and observation handed down from generation to generation whether verbally or in writing (Sofowora 1984; WHO 1976). In his view, Owumi (1993) while expatiating on the WHO conception of traditional medicine maintains that it is an art which is original and originates from the group, transmitted through time which is acceptable, triable affordable and accessible within the group where it obtains.

The impact of colonialism spread of western education and globalization of culture provided good horizons for certain alterations in the practices of traditional medicine. In this direction, it is not to say that traditional medicine has lost its potency and acceptability. As observed by writers on traditional medicine, 75% of Nigerian population still uses traditional medicine despite irreconcilable efforts of modern medicine to substantiate it (Sofowora 1983; Pearce 1986; Owumi 1993).

It is also noticed that economic crisis and political uncertainties affect many developing countries to have reinvented the popularity of traditional medicine. This is due to inability or difficulty of these countries to meet up with the requirements of importation of modern drugs, as the medical system is overcapitalized and sophisticated. Maternal and child healthcare is affected by the trends of change in medical practices in Nigeria. The changing pattern feature attempts at integrating traditional medicine with western medicine.

Authors have equally noticed that the practice of traditional system of MCH have some cultural factors which have significant effects both negatively and positively on MCH (Hyma and Ramesh 1994: 272). For instance, Tella (1977) declared that the use of Traditional Birth Attendants (TBAs) is promotive to MCH especially in the rural communities. Many other writers have pointed out some practices which are harmful to MCH. In her work, Odebiyi (1977) asserted that the use of contaminated concoction and cow dung and urine as traditional medicine are harmful.

Maternal Child Healthcare in Nigeria

Clearly affected by alteration in traditional medical system is the maternal and child healthcare system (MCH) in Nigeria. Most especially the child bearing period and the children under five are reputably faced with the risks of structural dualism and imbalance in Nigerian medical system (Aregbeyen 1988, 1991, 1994). Modern healthcare system shows dichotomy between the rural and urban healthcare system on one hand and between the rich and the poor on the other hand. The situation exposed the rural population to health problems such as lack of adequate facilities to have sustained western medical care system. The disparity between the poor and the rich with 75% of Nigerians falling below poverty level has exposed this larger population to health risks due to their inability to meet up with the cost of the services in western medicine. Sequel to these dichotomies and imbalances are the differential opportunities afforded to educated and uneducated individuals by modern healthcare system in the country. With more than 60% of the population still uneducated, more than half of the population could not enjoy the provisions of modern health facilities (Afonja 1996; Jinadu 1998, Owumi 2002).

It has also been noted that in view of high vulnerability of women and children to the heralded problems associated with the development of modern medicine in the developing countries, especially during pregnancy, childbirth and at infancy, attentions have been directed to Child Survival Initiative (CSI) and Safe Motherhood Initiative (SMI) (Price 1994; Smyke 1991; Williams Baumslang and Jeliffe 1989). However, these authors have indicated the trend in mortality rates in maternal and child health in their various writings. It is noted that out of 40,000 children who die annually, large concentrations are found in the developing societies without an exclusion of Nigeria. In 1990, the mortality rate for under five children ranged between 120 and 180 per 1,000 live births in most of the developing countries of the world. UNICEF and WHO have reported in different statistical records that between 1993 and 1996, mortality rates for mothers and children increased in the developing countries especially where there were political crises. In Nigeria, health indications revealed that infant mortality oscillated between 120 and 97 deaths per 1000 live births between 1993 and 2007. The health watch released by U.N. Population Data Sheet accounted for slight decrease in infant mortality to less than 100: 1000 live births in 1997 (UN Population Data Sheet 1997; UNICEF 1990, 1991, 1992, 1993, 1994, 1996; WHO 1998, 1992).

Other writers in this field have shown curiosities. Twaddle (1996) referred to this as resilient silent emergency and the neglected tragedy of child ill-health and maternal poor state of health respectively. In their works separately, Aregbeyen (1991) and Pearce (1986) expressed concerns on why it is impossible for the modern intervention to have stemmed the incidence of maternal and child mortality. They noted inherent problems in child health development programmes initiated in the country. In view of these curiosities, there is a need to examine various maternal and child health development programmes in Nigeria so as to bring out their flaws.

It is noted that 1970s saw an increased awareness of the importance of health and development in Nigeria focusing on mothers and children. This marked the beginning of new era in health. This attempt became necessary as it was realized that:

> The wholesale transfer of western style curative health care was failing to meet the needs of the majority of the people (Oyeneye 1985).

Thus, in Nigeria, the establishment of Basic Health Scheme Services (BHSS) in 1975-1980 third National Development Plan was witnessed. Although BHSS failed as a result of financial, manpower, political planning and implementation pitfalls (Oyeneye 1985; Ityanuyar 1987), yet it marked a change in approach to maternal and child healthcare from curative to preventive and much more to community based (Ajala 1995). Upon the recognition of these interests, the enunciation of Primary Health Care system (PHC) in 1985 with all-embracing strategies was to make the healthcare affordable, accessible and preventive-oriented (Oke 1993). PHC marked the introduction of Child Survival and Development Resolution (CSDR) encompassing Growth monitoring, oral rehydration therapy, breastfeeding and immunization, food supplements, family spacing and female education known under the acronyms of GOB I-FFF (Price 1994; Smyke 1991; Williams Baumslang and Jelliffe 1989).

However the above programmes did not meet the required success largely due to certain socio-cultural factors influencing children and mothers' health. One of these factors is mothers' educational status. According to Erinosho (1977), in Nigeria educated people are more likely to utilize western-style of healthcare services. He also noted that influence of magico-religious factors are less upheld on the conception of healthcare system among the educated people than non-educated people. More to this factor is the non-literates mothers have preference for traditional healing system than the literate mothers. This is because the official conducts in the hospital such as queuing for cards, registration, and physical examination are cumbersome, strange and seem alienating to non-literates.

Gender factor is also identified as a significant variable affecting maternal and child healthcare system. It is noted by Erinosho (1998) that women in some ethnic groups in Nigeria will not seek immediate help from healthcare agents until they obtain formal permission from their husbands. Some other women as a result of gender consciousness and religious attachment prefer to be examined by female physicians or health workers. So in the absence of their desires, they prefer to deliver babies at home where older women within their households assist in child-delivery. These attitudes are the outcomes of decision-making on health seeking that has interplay between education and illness as well as health behavior among women in the rural communities (Ajala 2000). Therefore, the bottom-line of all these arguments is that social status of the users has a dominant factor on the utilization and decision-making in healthcare system.

Family income is another important determinant factor in the pattern of utilization of healthcare institution as well as in the conception of healthcare system. Studies conducted by World Bank (1990) revealed that rural people are more likely to use traditional healing system not because of lack of health infrastructure, but mainly because of the perceived cost of modern health services which their income may not permit.

Another social factor which determines maternal and child healthcare delivery is the location of the health facilities. According to Coliver et al (1967), mothers and children would want to use clinics, which are nearer their homes. Studies on the relationship on spatial location and use of healthcare facilities show that patients are likely to utilize health services which are near to their normal abode than those which are farther away because of travel time, transport and other costs. Scholars like Okafor (1982) have significantly argued that proximity along with high incomes and participation in strenuous occupation are equally important determinants of healthcare delivery services.

Cultural Factors in MCH

From our understanding of culture, it is a basic assumption that children everywhere are born into two external worlds. The first is that of physical and geographical surroundings which according to Williams and Jelliffe (1982) may mean the specific environmental conditions into which the particular child is born. The second world is that of culture. That is the harmful or beneficial interconnected system of customs, ideas, attitudes, beliefs and behaviours that has been created for children before or soon after they are born by their mothers. As part of socialization, the rearing of the new born children revolves round cultural milieu.

In essence, the local cultural pattern is of great importance to MCH. Jelliffe and Bennett (1960) observed that these cultural patterns are important because it created to an understanding of cultural factors underlying disease patterns in the community. It also gives insight into people's values, knowledge of and attitude to health and disease. It may also enable scientific medicine to become enriched by new ideas, methods and techniques.

From the foregoing, cultural factors in MCH are the cultural patterns related to the practice of childbirth and rearing, which are either harmful or beneficial. Thus, from the array of literature reviewed so far, it is true that our knowledge of culture, medicine and traditional system of MCH have been espoused. Also, we have gained some practical knowledge on social and cultural factors in MCH. Nonetheless, the succinct idea, knowledge, practices and attitudes encompassing the practice of MCH in the rural communities are either lacking or remaining scanty in the existing literature. Also notable of good attention is the direction and analysis of change in health culture of the people. Previous writers have focused attention on incorporation approach of social change. Identification of these crucial issues in maternal and child healthcare provoked this study to examine social and cultural factors influencing the utilization of MCH services in rural communities of Osun State, to bring out the succinct ideas related to MCH in the rural areas. It also aimed at drawing attention to urgent need to refocus on our model of change. These are the gaps in the existing literature which this work fills.

4

Knowledge and Beliefs in MCH

Introduction

As noted earlier, the scope of maternal and child healthcare includes all practices undertaken towards the conception of human offspring, their birth, their caring between age zero and five as well as the health caring for the women under the childbirth age. Therefore in the foregoing, we shall examine the data gathered from the respondents as they relate to their knowledge, attitude, belief and practice of MCH in rural communities of Osun State.

Conception of MCH

At the onset, there is need to explain the word conception which is formed from concepts. Concepts are ideas or notions underlying a class of things. Despite the fact that there is a universal denominator to every concept, concepts still have peculiar meaning to specific people practicing them. For instance, according to World Health Organization (1978), health as a concept implies the general well-being other than absence of disease and deformity. In that wise, health implies social, economic, political and infrastructural comfort in human society. It is certain from the field investigation that not all human societies employ that index to measure their state of health.

Among the traditional Yoruba people, health implies a state of harmony between mind and the body (Jegede 1994). According to them, sickness implies all distasteful behaviours which include all anti-social behaviours. To be healthy therefore means a balance state of mind and body which embrace physical, mental and socio-biological well-beings. That is the state of "homeostasis". The traditional Yoruba conception of health does not include absence or inadequacy of infrastructure as reflected in WHO conception of health. Their conception does not reflect any reference to good roads, potable water and many other institutionalized agencies which are directly linked to good health.

All the respondents without formal education (almost 75 percent of our respondents) maintained that good or bad roads have nothing to do with good or bad health. They hold the view that health is pathological abnormality which is characterized by a set of symptoms and signs. The abnormality in fewer cases may be caused by infections. For instance, if one eats spoilt foods, and in a little more cases unripe fruits, exposed to poor weather, as in the case of somebody exposed to hot weather. Such person may have fever and malaria. But in more cases, disease to the traditional Yorubas especially in rural communities is caused by affliction from spiritual agents such as spirits of the dead, witchcraft, sorcerers and gods.

The community studied maintained that disease is any form of physical or spiritual problem which prevent someone from attending to his/her physical, social, economic and moral functioning, in a way the society has prescribed. It is anything which may cause malfunctioning and discomfort in the body system (Osunwole 1989). In these communities, diseases are variously referred to as *aisan* i.e. not well or *ailera* (not well) or *aare* (not sound), *amodi* (not well for a long time) or *ojojo* (not balanced). Regardless of linguistic variations, a slight distinction exists between illness and disease especially among the Igbominas and Oyo Yorubas. For instance, in Igbomina, iba (fever) especially malaria is not regarded as illness but as a disease, whereas, the Oyo regards malaria as illness. Illness is specifically referred to as *aare* that is a long time sickness. Disease is generally referred to as aisan (not well). The two terms are used interchangeably to refer to socio-biological misfit in individual. Thus, the two words are synonymous in most Yoruba conception of disease. In illness, the actor or actress may not be stopped in his or her physical engagements but certainly he/she would display certain abnormality in deviance to the community behavior. For instance, a child suffering from wasting or kwashiorkor is not having disease but he is only ill. Disease on the other hand is the complete breakdown of the body system. The two concepts have to do with poor state of health; while disease is the penultimate stage of poor health, illness though abnormal may be the starting point of poor health which is underrated by the people. Thus, a respondent when asked what killed her child responded:

> *Omo naa tie yami lenu, ko saisan rara o, o kan sere wala lati ile keji ni, o si sun mo mi lo ba n bi, o si n gbon, ka ti e to gbe dodo baba n sale, o ti ku.*

> I was surprised about the incidence, he was not sick at all. He just ran to the house from the neighbouring house and moved to me. He started vomiting and was shivering. Before I took him to Baba n sale (Baba n sale is a herbalist) he had died.

In a general term, both illness and disease are conditions of abnormal quality, unpleasantness of the mind, negative physical, social and moral quality, the absence of harmony between body and mind, troublesomeness, pain and discomfort (Jegede 1994, 1996). All the above conditions are capable of affecting all human beings, young and old, male and female. This suggests that keeping human beings safe of these infirmities; medical practices are essential aspects of culture. All these practices are health behaviors, which are enshrined in culture. All efforts required securing pregnancy, safe delivery and the survival of the mothers and children are cultural practices known as maternal and child healthcare (MCH) system. MCH system includes health-seeking practices aimed at securing the lives of the mothers and their children; pregnancy and childbirth process and household nutritional culture. It also includes childrearing practice and preparation for parenthood and household structures and relations. To fulfill the above requirements, the communities employ the service of traditional, western and faith healing. In these communities, there is practice of syncretism whereby two or more of the above healthcare systems are mixed.

Before the advent of European missionary and colonialism, health practices related to MCH were through indigenous medical system. The introduction of European missionary and colonialism saw the establishment of orthodox medical practices in Nigeria (Schram 1971). Although before the widespread of western orthodox medicine, there was a practice of Arabic brand of medicine which featured the inscription of some portions of Holy Quran on slates and being washed for drinking as medication.

With the introduction of colonialism in the early 19th century in Nigeria, a stage was gradually set for competition between indigenous and orthodox practices of MCH. In the rural communities which lacked adequate coverage by the missionaries, the predominant practices were the traditional methods of MCH. The urban locations saw the practice of western/orthodox practices. This practice was maintained during the independence era and shortly thereafter. Significantly in 1970s, socio-economic crisis faced by the country called for integration of indigenous and orthodox practices of maternal and child healthcare in Nigeria (Tella 1992). This approach was not a total success not until 1985 when Primary Health Care programme (PHC) began. The programme centres on healthcare for mothers and children, through community-oriented approach.

PHC was pursued vigorously between 1985 and 1993 when spirited attempts were made to immunize children and mothers against five deadly diseases, nutritional culture of the people was enhanced; Family Planning methods were introduced among other programmes. Through this programme (PHC), many health innovations were instituted.

Between 1993 and 1999, when the country faced harsh socio-political crises which affected its economy both at micro and macro levels, PHC programme was relaxed and the rural communities felt more brunt in the maternal and child healthcare. Although the programme still pursued immunizations, yet breakdown of health infrastructural facilities and loss of foreign supports by the government adversely affected the PHC programmes. As a result of these crippling situations, rural communities renewed their traditional system of maternal and child healthcare.

In rural communities of Osun state, 55.0% of the population prefers and utilize traditional method of maternal and child healthcare system. Starting from the conception of pregnancy, the pregnant woman is registered with the traditional healer who takes care of the pregnancy and the woman until and after delivery. Medication features concoction, offering sacrifice and ritual if the situation demands for it. Modern or orthodox health system which featured the institutionalized hospitals such as maternities, primary healthcare centers and in a serious health problem, secondary healthcare institutions may be used. The hospital setting shows permanent western-trained doctors. The third system is faith-healing predominant especially among the Christ Apostolic Church who has healing centers, which employ the use of prayer, holy water and divine oil in maternal and child healthcare. The fourth system which is also identified is syncretism. In syncretism, the patients combine two or more of the above systems in their healthcare practice.

The research finding shows that 55.0% of the respondents rely purely on traditional system while 17.1% of the respondents mix the three systems together. Only 20.2% relies on exclusive modern healthcare and 7.1% practices the faith-healing (see Table 2).

Table 2: Methods of Caring in MCH in Rural Communities of Osun State

Methods	No. Sampled (480)	%
Traditional	256	55.0
Modern	102	20.2
Faith-healing	34	7.1
syncretism	85	17.1

The above conception guides the treatment and caring of mothers and children during the maternal and child age among these rural Yorubas of Osun State.

Reluctance to patronize modern healthcare system is blamed on heavy charges and social status of the auxiliary health workers attached to those hospitals. A respondent said that *ako awon nurse yen ti e ti poju. Won ki ro wipe eniyan bi tiwon naa ni awa naa. Emi o lo be mo n temi o. Olorun lo n toju mi.* That is, "those nurses are too proud; they don't consider us as human beings like them. As for me, I am not going there again. I leave my health for my God". Location of the hospitals with poor road access is another inhibiting factor to the utilization of modern healthcare system as noted by many of the respondents.

Belief System in MCH

Emphasis on supernatural causation of diseases encourages the utilization of traditional medicine at the neglect of modern medicine. It is noted from the data that 55.0% of the respondents favor the use of traditional medicine (see Table 2 above). Traditional medicine is also predominantly favoured by many people using syncretism. Therefore, an aggregate of 72.1% of our respondents can be said to favor traditional medicine (17.1% for syncretism and 55.0% for pure traditional medicine).

Services for traditional medicine are provided by persons ascertained to have acquired the power of healing either at birth through inheritance or through specialized training. Traditional healers found in the research areas include the herbalists, diviners and *Elewe-omo* especially in Okinni. Usually, the herbalists are knowledgeable of efficacy of herbs to cure ailments while some diviners (*Baba-*

lawo) do not have deep knowledge of the use of herbs but they are consulted on the causes of diseases. They are also employed to undertake sacrifice and other related rituals for the patients. Those rituals may include animating the soul of the patients. However, there are still some other Babalawos who have both skill of divination and herbalism. The third category of traditional healers connected with MCH is *Elewe-omo*. *Elewe-omo* is the traditional specialists in pediatric nursing with the use of herbs. They can prescribe herbs for the mother to go and prepare for both the infants and mothers. These practitioners are mostly used than the other two.

The utilization pattern reflects the social status. While the literates prefer *Elewe-omo* if at all they want to use traditional medicine, the Babalawos and herbalists are more patronized by non-literates. Table 3 below shows the frequency of utilization of traditional medicine.

Table 3: Utilization Patterns of Traditional Medicine in MCH

Types of Trad. Medicine	Formal Education	%	Non-Formal Education	%
Diviners	3	11.5	62	66.5
Herbalist	7	26.9	7	7.4
Elewe-omo	16	61.5	25	26.5

From Table 3 above, a selected sample of 120 mothers who confessed using traditional medicine was obtained in all the research sites. Out of these 120 mothers, 26 of them were literates while 94 were non-literates. From their responses, it was revealed that 66.5% of non-literates use the diviners while 7.4% of the same category of mothers similarly employs the use of herbalists. Only 11.55 of literates who use diviners do so when the illness is protracted and bear the conception that supernatural causation is involved.

The respondents using traditional medicine generally advanced four reasons why they prefer the traditional medicine. The first reason is that the healers are more effective in some diseases such as convulsion, smallpox, measles and *Abiku*. All these diseases are believed to be outside the knowledge of western medicine. Another reason provided is that traditional medicine provides a greater psychological satisfaction which they claimed to be very impressively present in the mystical environment where the healers operate. Another set of our respondents believe that traditional medicine is cheap, affordable and available without any bureaucratic delay. They claimed that traditional healers can be paid installmentally. Also, a sizeable number of our respondents believes that they know all what the traditional healers use as medicine unlike the prepared drug in modern medicine whose compositions are unknown to the patients.

Belief in traditional healer is so strong that they are never considered failure. They are always successful, even if symptoms persist after being treated by traditional healers. Many other reasons other than the failure of traditional medicine are proffered. Such reasons may include the exposure of the medicine to the interference of weather conditions, failure of the patients to follow the prescribed conditions especially when the medicine includes incantation. Other factors may include disapproval of the treatment by the fate or destiny of the patient and that enemies have interfered with the medicine, then spoiling its efficacy.

The above belief is to establish the security of the reputation of the traditional healers. Belief in the efficacy of traditional healer has resulted in poor patronage of modern health facilities among the rural people of Osun State. The people find the traditional healers more convenient, readily accessible and more available. Another traditional healthcare feature prominently among the people is the use of Traditional Birth Attendants (TBAs). For instance in Ibodi, 65.4% of mothers with child delivery between 1998 and 2000 reported that they employed the services of TBAs. These TBAs are attached to maternity centers in the community and in Ilesha. In other research sites, the record is not as high as what obtained in Ibodi, yet there is none of our research sites where the record is lower than 48.2%.

Following an in-depth interview held on the reason for the high patronage of TBAs in the research areas. Fifty-three percent (53.4%) of the women that delivered babies between 2005 and 2007 in all the studied communities agreed that the TBAs show continued interest in the welfare of the baby. The TBAs consider those babies as theirs and the babies enjoy deep affections from the TBAs. Another reason provided by 39.4% of our key informants on TBAs was that the TBAs provide alternative to going to a distant hospital and as such, in emergency situation, the TBAs are better preferred. The remaining 7.2% claimed that TBAs are mothers with rich experience in child delivery. They are verse in handling deliveries and their cost is cheaper, reasonable and affordable. The high patronage of these TBAs shows that they are neighborhood institution who identify with their patients at little or no cost.

Apart from the above variables, religious affiliation also has influence on the utilization of maternal and child healthcare services in the rural communities of Osun State. There are three religious groups identified in the research area. These are the Muslims, Christians and Traditional religions. Among the Muslims, the belief in plural marriage is upheld and common. Thus, the family size is always large. Some of these Muslims also practice pudah (woman-in-seclusion). The practice of pudah amongst these Muslims tends to lower patronage of maternity centres. These Muslims hardly utilize maternal and health childcare services, except when it has become unavoidable. These rural Muslims also do not want to go against the decision of their husbands since they are kept in pudah, they engaged in petty trading which earns very little incomes for them. Since the practice is polygyny, husbands have little concern for the maternal and child needs of the family. As a result of all these factors, they resort to the use of faith-healing and quoranic medicine. This includes Muslim prayer and inscription of quoranic verses on tabloid which they wash and drink as medicine. There is none of the maternal and infant diseases which are incurable to them. There is also the practice of syncretic medicine which feature the use of herbs combined with quoranic medicine for mothers and children.

A similar situation occurs among the Christian sect of Aladuras and Christ Apostolic Church (CAC). Among these sects, the use of the word of God according to the Bible, holy water and anointing oil together with prayer and fasting are common. In Okinni and Tonkere, there are maternity centres being operated by C.A.C where all these medical therapies are used. In these maternity centres, patients are admitted. These maternity centres are managed by the church leaders who could either be a male as in Tonkere or female as in the case of Okinni. They claimed to have been trained in maternal and child health caring in conformity to the principles of Apostolic Church. Other Christian sects adopt the use of modern health facilities or sometimes engage in syncretism.

The traditional religious practitioners favour the use of various traditional systems of MCH. Eighty-five percent of our respondents who are traditional religious practitioners do not engage in any other MCH system other than either the TBAs, herbalists or the diviners. The remaining 15% engage in plural medicine of traditional and modern health system for mothers and children.

5

Social and Economic Factors in MCH

Customs and Habits Associated with MCH

There exist a wide range of customs and habits associated with maternal and child healthcare in the rural communities of Osun State. These have considerable influence on the health of both mothers and their children. While some of these customs and habits have good effects on MCH, most of them are dangerous to the health of mothers and children.

The practice of intensive and prolonged breastfeeding among this rural people at least for up to one year or over affords them the opportunity of birth control. It is believed that during breastfeeding, menstruation is delayed and ovulation is inhibited, therefore the likelihood of conception is drastically reduced (Isuigo-Abanihe and Iloh 1999). Among this people, 68.2% of mothers confirmed the practice of prolonged and intensive breastfeeding for a period of at least a year. During this period, there is sexual abstinence which often lasted than the period of lactation or weaning of the child.

This practice is upheld through the common belief that a sexually active breastfeeding woman opens her child to problem of sucking semen, which they thought, can mix with the breast milk and contaminate the milk. They believe that such can cause diarrhea and wasting as well as stunted growth in children. The result supposedly is infant mortality. Mothers similarly believed that long period of sexual abstinence after birth is also considered necessary to ensure the health of mothers and children. The community views some women who failed to observe this tradition negatively. Reports showed that a new pregnancy has effect on the health of the sucking child. Therefore, the traditional belief is that sexual relations during the period of breastfeeding are socially proscribed for a period that may vary from several months to several years after the birth of a child. The implication of the above practice is that it added to the birth interval when it extends longer than postpartum infecundity.

Similarly, the prevalence of fresh fruits and vegetables in the localities provides food supplements to loss food calories due to food prejudices and taboo. The people especially children have rich intake of fresh fruits and vegetable which provide them with essential minerals and other micronutrients' requirements for their growth. Fruits such as oranges, pineapples, pawpaw, cashews, guava, banana and plantain are common at little or no cost. So, the population derives food supplements from these fruits.

One of the customs and habits which is harmful to children is the use of forced feeding which is prevalent among this particular Yoruba people. This practice feature the use of water, maize gruel or any liquid, poured into the mothers' folded hand. During the process, the child cries and half-breathed with the food residues splash into the side of the child's face. The process also features the child been pinioned across the mothers' knees with his head downward. During this process, choking always occurs and the feed may even pass into the respiratory tract, which may result into respiratory infection. This method of feeding is prevalent among the rural women to the extent that it is practiced by 78.6% of the nursing mothers. This is a traditional practice which is resilient especially among the non-formal educated Yoruba women resident in traditional rural communities. The belief is that children don't like to eat unless they are forced. Some women similarly acclaimed that since children cannot express satisfaction directly, they have to be fed to show in them that they are well-fed. As a result of this, a mother becomes delighted seeing her baby's stomach bulged out. Mother can only achieve this through forcefully feeding their children, which does not take much time for the babies to be overfed.

Also, in some cases especially when meat is to be fed into the children, the rural women practice "tongue feeding" whereby meat item is chewed into paste by mothers or into pulp before it is transferred into children's mouth. Apart from the fact that this practice facilitates the spread of germs and infections, it is also noted that during the chewing of the items into paste, the nutritional values might have been digested and absorbed in the mouth of the mothers; hence, transferring roughage for the children.

Similarly, there are some nutritional practices which are harmful to child health security such as food discrimination. There are some food items which are not fed into children. Food items like egg, sugar, meat, groundnut cake are considered harmful to children. Ninety-eight percent (98.2%) of mothers interviewed believed that these food items are unfit for children. They believe that sugar and any other sweet objects such as honey cause diarrhea and pile *jedijedi*, while meat causes worm. Egg and groundnut cake are thought to make the child become a thief later in life. Some still believe that plantain and pepperish dishes are indigestible. The implication of this food taboo is the prevention of children from eating certain foods that are essential for their healthy growth. This prevents the success of food security services associated with MCH programmes.

The belief in children's power of reincarnation to torment their mothers also reigns supreme among the people studied. Children with this preter-natural power are known as *Abiku* are believed to defy all caring. The woman who suffers incessant infant mortality is believed to have been afflicted with *Abiku* spirit. Hence, there is little or nothing to do to prevail on this mortality. It is further believed that the traditional healers do not always have potency to cure this type of children. Hence, the Yoruba adage *Abiku sologun deke*, meaning "Abiku betrays herbalists", is always referred to in such cases. The belief is that these particular children having such power die soon after birth and reconceived to be born and die soonest. To check this, traditional rural women result to burning or mutilating the corpse of the victim. This preconceived idea prevents taking such children to hospital. The infantile death associated with *Abiku* is probably due to sickle cell haemoglobinopathy, which is common in the traditional Yoruba community. Many Yoruba people did not have in depth enough scientific understanding of its management, according to an auxiliary health worker's observation during the fieldwork.

There is also the problem of adolescent childbirth which is prevalent in the community studied. This problem also constitutes health hazards to both the adolescent mothers and their children. This problem always arises as a result of illicit and unprotected sex among the school girls (Ajala 2002). The practice was prevalent in Ibodi, where about 9.3% of our respondents (mothers) claimed that they were between 15 and 16years old when they were impregnated. Immediately the parents knew, they forced them to their suitors without even collecting bride pay. Since then they had become mothers. As at the time of research, many of these victims have had between three and four children each with the oldest among these mothers being 22years old. About 18% of the women interviewed entered into motherhood when they were between 15 and 20 years of age. This practice is too dangerous. In the first instance, all the reproductive organs might have not developed properly at this age, thus such habit result into complication at childbirth, which was reported to have claimed the lives of many mothers. Another dangerous childbirth age is women at 40 years still in motherhood. About 4.3% of our respondents (mothers) fall into this category. As indicated in table 4 below, about 23% of mothers are vulnerable to serious childbirth problems due to under-age and old-age. Childbirth at old age exposes women to hard labor in child delivery, which the body system may not likely sustain. Such may lead to various maternal health problems.

Table 4: Age at Childbirth (Women)

AGE RANGE	NO. OF WOMEN (N=480)	%
15 – 20	85	17.8
21 – 30	275	57.3
31- 40	95	19.8
41 – 50	20	4.2

The problem of childbirth at old age is usually due to divorce. When a woman divorces, she is still expected to bear children for the new husband to justify his investment on the new wife; and more importantly for the woman to be qualified to share in the new husband's property. It can also be as a result of infertility and the practice of widow inheritance following the death of an initial husband.

For fear of ridicules, the adolescent and old-age pregnant women though exposed to various health risks, do not always want to utilize MCH services. They either patronize quack doctors or employ self-medication which makes them vulnerable to complication and maternal mortality.

Method of rearing babies whose mothers die during labour constitutes another problem. Among these people, the practice is to foster the baby to relatives who are usually "retired" mothers and non-lactating. Such "mothers" will then artificially induce lactation. Method used to lactate includes putting the baby's mouth on the breast nipple to suckle and extract breast milk by force. If the milk is produced, it is of low calories. In some cases, it takes long time before the milk is produced. Such incidence results to starvation in children and capable of causing marasmus according to an auxiliary health worker interviewed as our key informant. Associated with this custom is the belief that such children stand a very slim chance of survival, so little efforts are given to their caring.

Generally, the practice of child fostering by the grandparents is prevalent among the rural people in Yoruba society. This practice features fostering children between age three and five to grandparents. The grandparents usually have delights in seeing their grandchildren, but lack enough skill and money to give them adequate care. Constituting more danger is the habit of these grandparents to foster grandchildren from each of their own children, thereby further deteriorating their already old age health (Ajala 2007). Such fostered children do not live in good and hygienic environment and lack basic care, thus resulting into child morbidity such as stunted growth and kwashiorkor which are capable of resulting to child mortality.

The practice of quack doctors is common in these rural communities. Ninety-seven percent of our respondents attested their use of quack doctors. These quack doctors are residents in all these communities and receive high patronage. The rural people are aware of their hazards, but still prefer them to qualified doctors. They call them different names such as *Koso n'gbo* which suggests that they are illegal. Their high patronage is blamed on non-availability of qualified doctors in all the research communities. As at the time of research, there was no qualified doctor in all these communities, either private or public. Even in the primary health and maternity centers available, there were only auxiliary health workers. The rural people therefore could not afford going to nearby urban settlement where qualified doctors were mostly present. Also encouraging the patronage of quack doctors is the lack of good access roads to urban locations. Only Ibodi and Telemu have good roads to Ilesha and Iwo respectively. Yet, in these areas likewise other communities, people still prefer the use of quack doctors because of their cheaper cost. Quack doctors can still allow payment of their charges installmentally. They are also preferred because they are accessible to the people at the rural communities. This practice is hazardous to the health of both mothers and children. Quack doctors are untrained doctors who have little or no knowledge about maternal and child healthcare. They operate on their patients under trial and error.

Closely related to this is the practice of self-medication in maternal and child healthcare. All the respondents claimed to have been involved in the practice. They claimed that they got the knowledge of drug prescription from their personal experience. Their experiences are gathered from friends or by themselves in their previous visits to hospitals. All these communities have unauthorized chemists who patronize them. They come from the urban centers to sell drugs for the rural people. Associated problems to this practice include overdose and drug abuse which may lead to complication in treatment of health problem.

Some health workers in the maternity centres affirmed that they always notice the use of quack doctors and self-medications on some patients who are at last taken to the hospital after such might have worsened the patients' case. This suggests that when quack doctor discovered themselves as incompetent to revive such patients, they referred the patients to hospitals. Many of such cases eventually resulted into mortality especially in children and women at child labor. Specifically, the practice of self-medication and quack doctors prevent the people from using the maternal and child healthcare services.

The practice of extra-marital sexual relationship, although highly reduced in the rural communities is another habit which is hazardous to maternal and child healthcare. Such may result to divorce even when the mother is still rearing children. In such occasion, the children are exposed to empty-cell family, where they are not adequately taken care of. The fear of ridicule has drawn some other women to go for unsafe abortion from the available quack doctors. Such cases often result to maternal mortality. This practice may also lead to transmission and spread of Sexually Transmitted Diseases (STDs). Despite the susceptibility to health hazards which this practice portends, the fear of ridicules and embarrassment discourages people affected from utilizing MCH services.

Poverty and Its Effects on MCH

Poverty, which has been considered as a broad concept that encompasses many aspects of life including social and physical environment, is indeed another major determinant of poor utilization of maternal and child healthcare services in the rural communities of Osun State. More so, holistic manifestation of poverty in these rural communities has greatest impacts on the environment, health related infrastructures, dietary intake of the people, the therapeutic choice of the patients and cumulatively on the maternal and child morbidity and mortality. It is shown that there are more diseases inflicted as a result of poverty of resources than those caused by germs and infections.

Socio-demographic information indicates that 75.3% of our male respondents are below poverty line while almost 75% of the female respondents are similarly below the poverty line of ₦3,000 earning per month, an equivalent of $30 per month.

Health problem emanating from poverty includes the inability of the population to provide much needed foods to support the increasing population in the
household due to higher rate, thus affecting food security aspect of MCH services. More importantly, the rural population lacks the economic power to revital-
ize their subsistence resources such as land and tools. Putting more pressure on
the health of these rural people is long periods of poor governance in Nigeria, a
situation that was characterized by corruption and state failure to provide adequate infrastructure for the people. Governance in Nigeria was also characterized by international debt burden, wrong and inequitable allocation of resources
as evidenced in perennial corruptions perpetrated by government officials and
long regimes of military governments which foreclosed possible international
assistance.

Cumulatively, all the above have serious effect on the utilization pattern of
MCH services especially the rural communities where the brunt was hardly felt.
In the first instance, military government and corruption in government pre-
vented the healthcare institutions from having adequate facilities which in turn
discouraged both the users and health workers. The users (patients) do not have
confidence on the service.

The poor economic status of the rural people was also associated with de-
clining agricultural production, industry and manufacturing which begun since
1980s. To alleviate these problems, the national government approached the International Financial Institutions (IFIs) for various loans on various terms which
further crippled the health of the people. These IFIs especially World Bank and
International Monetary Funds introduced harsh economic programmes which
the rural economy could not sustain (Ajala, 1999). The implication of these policies reflected in neglect of vital health policies and programmes such as Basic
Health and Social Scheme (BHSS) which was introduced in 1980s, to the favor
of more western-oriented health policies and programmes.

The introduction of Primary Health Care in 1985 was a watershed as a programme to alleviate poverty induced problems on healthcare of the people. Principally, maternal and child healthcare at the rural communities received greater
boost under PHC. The programme saw the introduction of expanded immunization programmes against six deadly diseases, that is, cholera, diphtheria, whooping cough, tetanus, marasmus and poliomyelitis. It was also designed to solve
maternal health problems such as complication at childbirth, unsafe pregnancy,
malnutrition and malaria, which has hitherto been affecting mothers and children especially in the rural communities.

Osun State was one of the States in Nigeria which received the pilot operation of Primary Health Care (PHC). Incidentally too, three of the communities
currently under study were chosen as pilot operation centers of PHC programmes in Osun State. These are Okinni in Egbedore Local Government, Ibodi
in Ilesha Local Government and Telemu in Ayedaade Local Government.

The gains of PHC were short-lived when as from 1990s, socio-political problems which are still the manifestation of resilient poverty, crippled the operation
of PHC in the country. Adversely affected by this sudden change are the rural
people who are the drawers of water and hewers of trees. Making the impact
more severe is their low level of literacy and rise in population at 3.2% annually.

The burden of poverty is physical on maternal and child healthcare services
of the rural people and it manifests in many forms. It shows on poor housing,
poor environmental sanitation and poor water supply. Due to poverty, women
and children are exposed to poor housing, which could not guarantee their health
security. They also lack access to good quality water. In Ekusa, reliance is on
streams for water. The stream is equally used for washing and swimming and
the people do not believe that such source for water could be polluted. A woman
respondent in Ekusa claimed that *egbin odo ki payan*. That means water pollu-
tion does not kill human being. She also alleged that people bath in the stream
and the stream still serves the community as drinking water. All these have direct impact on sustainable health programmes of the rural people of Osun state.
There is also uncontrolled vector occurrence, unemployment and underemploy-
ment, low educational achievement, poor access to health services and high
morbidity and mortality rate. Also, poverty has caused low production and lack
of political will to allocate necessary resources for social services and lack of
resources for social services, which eventually resulted into decline in infrastructures.

The resounding consequence of all this spiral course is the low socio-
economic status of women which imposes heavy burdened roles on them and
weaken their decision-making power on Reproductive and Family Healthcare
(RFH) especially in the areas of maternal and child healthcare system.

Women Social Roles and Effects on MCH

One of the underlying effects of poverty in the rural communities of Osun State
is low production affecting women's status. This exposes women to a lot of
strenuous activities which have cumulative effects on their health and that of
their children.

Women in these rural communities are saddled with lot of functions vis-à-vis
domestic functions. They prepare food and domestic needs of the family. Such
include the fetching of water usually from far distant places. They also engage in
economic activities such as farming which is hard. In Ekusa most women engage in traditional soap making and in Okinni, they are engaged in frying of garri. In Ibodi and Tonkere, many women engage in palm kernel cracking and
palm-oil refinery. All these works are strenuous as they were operated with manual labor. During these strenuous works, they still contend with caring for their
children and other associated reproductive activities for the family. In many occasions, these women create less time on childcare especially when they are at

the crucial stage in these works. Many of them whose husbands are farmers compulsorily help their husbands in farm work.

The effects of these social roles are indirectly noticed on maternal and child healthcare in these rural communities. Women have little or no time to attend hospitals. They are also not available for household health education and other related programmes such as Expanded Programmes on Immunization (EPI). Also, as a result of these social roles, children are neglected during work. During that time, the practice is that such children are given little or no attention.

6

Rural Health Care and MCH in Osun state

Various health statistical indexes reflect maternal and infant mortality rate in Nigeria as high (UN Population Data Sheet 1999). Infant mortality between 1996 and 1998 was put between 191 deaths/1000 live births and 110 deaths per 1000 live births in Nigeria. Maternal mortality is also between 110 and 100 deaths per 1000 women. It has also been reported that more than 75% of this mortality occurs at the rural communities as a result of preventable diseases.

Due to inadequate record on mortality in the rural communities, it is difficult to quantify the exact mortality rate in the research area. It is however obvious that maternal and infant mortality affects these rural communities of Osun State. High mortality rate in children especially the under 5, are primarily due to preventable and communicable diseases and poor nutrition, which are reflections of poverty-stricken rural communities.

In the communities studied, the seven top causes of death in children of under five are:

1) Malaria
2) Diarrhea related diseases
3) Acute respiratory diseases
4) Infectious and parasitic diseases such as cholera, tuberculosis and whooping cough.
5) Prenatal infections which includes low birth weight and malnutrition during pregnancy.
6) Nutritional disorders such as underweight and kwashiorkor, stunting and wasting.
7) Other deadly diseases including neo-natal tetanus, diphtheria and poliomyelitis (Ministry of Health Record, Osun State).

Against the maternal health care are the complication of childbirth, malnutrition during pregnancy and hemorrhage. Data on mortality and morbidity against maternal and child healthcare reflect three patterns of causation. These are:

1) Underlying factors
2) Intermediate factors
3) Direct factors

From the figure 3 below, the underlying factors are the potential and inherent cultural attitudes and behaviours which are capable of generating intermediate causes. The intermediate factors are those factors which can lead to direct factors. The first major factors accounted for maternal and child mortality and morbidity are the underlying factors. These factors include: women social status, cultural food prejudices, gender discrimination, maternal depletion syndromes, poverty, harmful traditional practices and many other cultural factors.

Second factors are the intermediate factors which only feature the utilization patterns of MCH development programmes. Determinants of these factors are acceptability, availability, and vulnerability, quality of care, accessibility and logistics. All these are the constructs of health decision-making.

The third factors are enshrined as direct factors. These are malnutrition, infection, illicitly induced abortion, childbirth complication, diarrhea, six deadly diseases and accidents.

Immediate Factors   Intermediate factors

Women social status;
Food Prejudices;
Gender discrimination;
Maternal depletion;
Poverty; and Harmful
traditional practices.

Acceptability and,
availability of healthcare
systems; Vulnerability
to diseases; Quality and
logistics involved in
care system. Infant and
Maternal Morbidity and
Mortality

Direct Factors

Malnutrition; Infec-
tions; Induced /Illicit
abortion; Child birth
complications; Diarr-
hea; and the six deadly
diseases.

Effects

Child and Maternal
morbidity and
mortality.

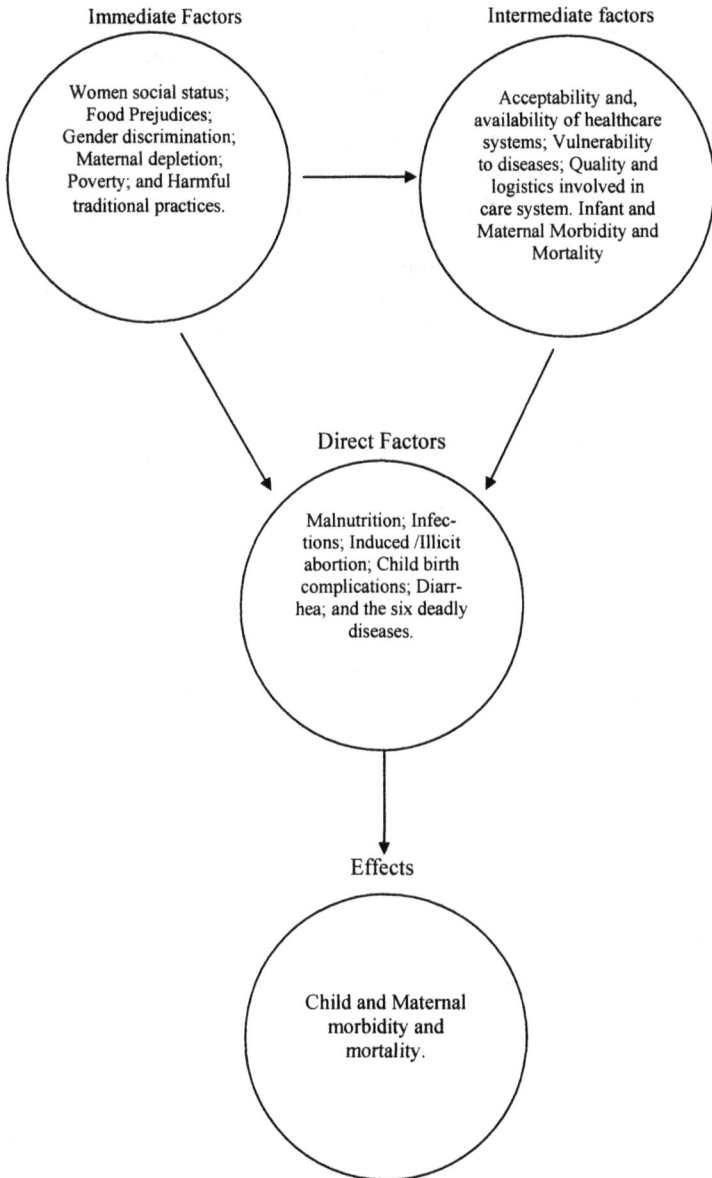

Figure 3: Causes of Maternal and Child Mortality and Morbidity
in Rural Communities of Osun State, Nigeria.

There is an interaction among the above mentioned three layers of causality of morbidity and mortality in MCH, through: (i) cultural and social practices; (ii) Health care planning and (iii) Disease and illness. The immediate factors are instances in cultural and social practices that inform health decision making. If these practices are negative, coupled with poor health care planning by the authorizing agencies, the intermediate factors turn negative. The outcomes are the list of direct factors which in turn leads to child and maternal morbidity and mortality.

Since rural health care provisioning in Osun state especially between 1980 and 2008 remained unfriendly to the rural population, there existed negative cultural and social practices and attitudes that prompted negative factors. These interactions in turn led to the onset of direct factors- diseases and illness causing high rate of MCH mortality.

7

Conclusion

From the foregoing, it is obvious that all communities, despite the degrees of technical sophistication, urbanization and industrialization have evolved their different cultural patterns which can be defined as the common way of life shared by all members of the group. These common, but specific practices include the preferred life goals, their valued ends and sanctioned means and their attitudes towards life and death (Williams and Jelliffe 1978), but also all aspects of their medical life, everyday life and the relationships between different members of a family. It also includes the traditional ways of doing things which include the preparation of foods and rearing of children as well as the modern and most recently approved methods of getting the lives fulfilled.

The above suggests that the cultural patterns of a group of people are subsumed on learnt behaviors which are partly acquired by deliberate instructions of the older members, but mostly absorbed subconsciously by incidental observation of behavior of relatives and other close members of the community. This process of learning begins at birth and in most cases even before the birth, and mediated by every contact the infant has with the surrounding world. This includes, for example, the ways the young children are cared, the roles of the parents and community both of the immediate contact and distant, and concepts that become habitual and customary, the food that are or are not eaten within a particular community. So also, the social, economic and political policies and programmes initiated by the institutional authorities. The overall actions of the community that is, mothers, fathers and children to all these patterns are the contents of reproductive and family health (RFH) which maternal and child health (MCH) is its integral part.

There are five aspects of cultural patterns which are of particular and direct relevance to maternal and child healthcare in the rural communities studied. These are:-
1) Indigenous Medical Systems
2) Mating, Pregnancy and Childbirth
3) Household Nutritional Culture
4) Child rearing Practice and Preparation for Parenthood and
5) Structures of Household and Household Relations.

All these are the broad factors having effects on rural health care provisioning in Osun state. If they are in positive positions, they are beneficial to the security and survival of mothers and children in the rural communities. However, if in negative position, they are harmful and capable of having deleterious effect on the rural management of MCH.

As observed in this work, the continuous practice of indigenous medicine suggests that the practice is adaptive and continues to meet the health needs of the rural people. The conception of health and culture is even traditional; therefore, the approach to health care security should not be totally divorced from this tradition. In traditional practice of MCH among these rural people, there are certain salient practices which are beneficial to the health security of people. So also, these practices need incorporation into modern practices. Such incorporation should be integrated into the entire cultural background and conceptions of the people to ensure positive change and development in the area of MCH. Therefore, it is opined that a rethinking of social change model is needed. In this direction, our approach of analyzing and studying social change should not be confined to incorporation approach but certainly we need a refocusing. Firstly, the community of the planned change must first witness transformation. The process here includes enlightenment and setting good socio-economic background for the change to be introduced. Therefore, instead of incorporation, integration should be the focus. That is blending the guest culture with transformed hosting culture. This in essence, is transformatory-integrational model in the adoption of innovation. Integration of some useful traditional practices should be done in this manner with the modern practices.

This becomes very imperative from our understanding of culture, that no culture is perfect. In every culture, there are both harmful and beneficial patterns. For instance, in the field of child health among different socio-economic groups; in Britain, over-rigid attitudes towards toilet training and the regularities of infant feeding; the use of proprietary "gripe-water" types of medicines and potentially dangerous mercurial "teething powders", the belief that fish is a specific "brain food" for infants are all cultural patterns which may constitute harmful practices. This is because all these related practices have been discovered to have harmful effects on child rearing in that society. There are more wide ranges of fad and superstitions, some old such as unnecessary over feeding of young babies with semi-solid and the exaggerated reliance on packaged and processed foods which are also of little benefit to MCH in Britain. Although many households in Britain are beginning to abandon all or some of the above mentioned fads, yet as it has not being totally eradicated, it is still part of MCH practices in the society. The point here is that it is important to recognize the cultural absurdities in one's own culture and particularly to prevent unwitting and harmful export in health education. The ill-effects of a particular custom may then be modified while at the same time, the essence of a culturally accepted practice is retained.

Once again, the fact here is that the observance of tradition, even if they are apparently unnecessary or "irrational" helps people to identify with their family or community. Such practices may form a cardinal factor in social development and stability. One may assume that it is as a result of many developed countries withdrawal from such observance that has called for a new focus on indigenous knowledge practices.

Sudden change witnessed in Yoruba traditional medical system especially during the colonial periods up to the late 70s, has greatly affected the indigenous practice of MCH in the community. As noted above, such sudden change was caused by internationalization of culture especially as in the spread of western education. Hence, western medical system was introduced and gained more acceptances against the traditional system until the 1970s. This situation exposed the rural people to structural dualism and imbalance in the medical system. Modern healthcare system reflects dichotomies between rural and urban healthcare; the rich and the poor and literates and illiterates. The cumulative effect is leaving 75% of Nigerian population who are below poverty line and resident in rural communities without access to literacy and vulnerable to severe attack in their maternal and child care system.

It has been noted above that more vulnerable are the women and children in the rural communities. To alleviate these problems, between 1970 and 1990, various health programmes were initiated which received both moral and financial boosts from both international agencies and national frontiers. Firstly in 1970s, the introduction of Basic Health and Social Scheme witnessed community participation in healthcare (Schram 1971). This scheme was designed to improve the quality of lives especially in the rural areas.

Between 1985 and 1990, primary health care was in operation with more focus on rural healthcare system. Its programmes were directed towards Child Survival and Development Revolution (CSDR), which encompassed growth monitoring, Oral Rehydration Therapy (ORT), breastfeeding and immunization, food supplements, family spacing and female education (GOBI-FFF) (Price 1994). This new approach saw a change from curative approach of healthcare system to preventive approach. To further strengthen the PHC programmes, there was a call for collaboration from traditional medicine, although unsuccessful as a result of cynism from modern health workers. Similarly too, the rural participation of Traditional Birth Attendants and provisions of health care facilities such as PHC centres in each local government secretariat in the country is a boost to PHC.

However, as laudable as the PHC programmes were, the gains were put into plunge as from 1993 when the country entered into a deep macro-economic decline and political crisis caused by the then military regimes. The effect of this was a drawback in the progress of PHC. The policy monitoring failed and the provided facilities entered into decay. Hard burden of international debt problem began to show on the health of the people especially the maternal and child healthcare in the rural communities. The situation continues with the increasing rate of maternal morbidity and mortality until 1999 when Nigeria reintroduced democratic governance, thus having a hope of revitalizing PHC programmes, which is yet to be done as at the time of writing.

In Osun State, the government has launched free medical services and integrated rural development since December 1999. All these were meant to empower the rural poor people so as to guarantee their health security. Also the federal government is committed to National Rebirth Programmes focusing on poverty alleviation action and rural development. Still, none of these new programmes was yet to have significant impact on the maternal and child healthcare of the rural people. This suggests that introduction of health care facilities is not enough to improve the health condition of a community. Also, imperative in health care strategy is the health decision which hinges on certain cultural factors.

Health decision of a particular set of people does not exclude their cultural factors. This implies that perception of one's health and the utilization of the available health facilities are governed by certain behaviours, habits and customs. Conceptions of health determine specific customs and habits generated towards securing the health of such population. As noted above, response to health challenges of the people may generate different classifications of customs and habits; which may be beneficial or harmless; uncertain and harmful. For instance, the prolonged breastfeeding among these rural people is beneficial as cultural family planning device. Similarly, faith-healing in MCH is an uncertain habit which possibly can be beneficial and harmful. This practice may not be opposed until further anthropological investigations are carried out. Certainly, it may be prejudicial and ethnocentric to assume that such practice is hazardous.

In the foregoing analysis, an examination of socio-cultural factors affecting maternal and child healthcare system in the rural communities of Osun State reveals the existence of a lot of socio-cultural factors affecting MCH especially in the rural areas, which still require an intensive research. For instance, women social roles and the practice of exclusive faith-healing in maternal and child healthcare require further investigation to establish their actual implication on the health security of both the mothers and children.

It is obvious that there are still in existence a lot of problems which hamper the safety of mothers and their children especially in the rural communities.

Policy Implications of the Study

In order to combat the problems of maternal and child morbidity and mortality especially in the rural communities, the living standard of the Nigerian population must first be raised. Extreme poverty of the people is not only the source of disease and mortality, but it is also one of the chief causes of bottlenecks in public health delivery in Nigeria, especially in the rural communities.

Maternal and child healthcare is a multi-sectoral system which calls for multi-sectoral approaches in its problem solving. On one hand, there is need for the social empowerment of women to have decision power in reproductive and family health. On the other hand, more attention should be directed to female literacy. In this approach, there is also a need for revitalization of agricultural production which is the basis of rural subsistence. If agricultural productivity is improved at household level, there will be more foods for the increasing population. In essence, the population policies must promote more equitable economic development and improved access to education, health and family planning services should be linked and integrated. For instance, breastfeeding must be promoted through MCH programme to help delay the resumption of ovulation, thus favoring pregnancy spacing and good maternal health.

In the same direction, traditional food crops are often consumed by rural people. A nutrition-focused agricultural policy that will boost rural production of these food supplies must be encouraged. This will help raise the rural income and at national level reduce demand for imported food.

Environmental degradation has a major impact on the health and nutrition of the rural people. The search for fuel wood takes an increasingly heavy toll on rural women's time and energy. Therefore, particular attention must go to developing sustainable production systems and rural technologies must be updated. Policy makers must recognize that the rural people are often forced to overexploit natural resources in order to survive. Therefore, environmental policies should aim at helping to increase access to resources and technologies especially in the rural communities. Harmful practices are main sources of concern in MCH and require modification by friendly persuasion in form of personal or group discussion and convincing demonstration of acceptable system subject to scientific verification. This can be done through health education and cultural integration.

On the direct intervention strategies, the current democratic governance should be sustained at all cost so as to have a review of Nigerian national health policy. Such new health policy should reflect adequate health promotion strategies such as provision of balanced infrastructural facilities including electricity, pipe-borne water, good roads and other health facilities at the rural communities. A well-articulated and strong political commitment to health promotion can only be guaranteed in democratic governance. Adequate funding of health services in Nigeria is also a well-deserving strategy. Maternal and child healthcare is a programme that has immense impact on general health of the people; hence its proper funding is a genuine course.

Finally, there is need for revitalization of Primary Health Care (PHC) in Nigeria. PHC is a fundamental means of responding to the community's need for health services. It ensures community participation in planning and implementing their own healthcare, generating health awareness, mobilizing the community and preventing infections. PHC is highly adaptive in maternal and child healthcare. On the whole, the integrated attention is a deserving solution to maternal and child health problems in the rural communities of Nigeria.

Bibliography

Adetunji, J.A, 1995. "Infant Mortality and Mothers Education in Ondo State, Nigeria", *Social Science and Medicine*, 40 (2): 1432-1447.

Ajaka Nji, 2004. *Why Poor People Remain Poor*. Yaoundé, DeSholar Press.

Ajala, A.S., 1995. "Some Associated Cultural Practices Related to Breastfeeding and Their Implication on Maternal and Child Health Care in Osun State, Nigeria". Unpublished M.A. Thesis at Institute of African Studies, University of Ibadan, Ibadan.

Ajala, A.S., 1999. "IMF Involvement in Nigerian International Debt Management: A Legal Analysis", An Unpublished Thesis at the Faculty of Law, Obafemi Awolowo University, Ile-Ife.

Ajala, A.S., 2000. "Socio-cultural Perspectives of Women's Health in Rural Communities of Osun State"; A Paper Delivered at the National Conference of Nigerian Anthropological and Sociological Association, O.A.U., Ile-Ife, 15th-16th November, 2000.

Ajala, A.S., 2000. Factors Affecting the Education of Adolescents' Sexual and Reproductive Health Rights in Rural Communities of Osun State, Nigeria". *Journal of Science Research*, 6 (2): 86-92.

Ajala, A.S., 2001. "Cultural Contexts of Inter-ethnic Relations before the Yoruba and Nupe Peoples in Ibadan City".In Igbie Ifie (ed.) *Papers in Honour of Prof. Tekenna Tamuno at 70* . Ibadan, Otuporo publisher, 27-42.

Ajala, A.S., 2007. "HIV/AIDS in Yoruba Perspectives: A Conceptual Discourse". *Journal of Social Sciences*, 14 (3): 235-241.

Ake, Claude, 1981. *The Political Economy of Africa*. London, Longman Press.

Akintoye Seith, 1995. "African Can Break Away from Diseases", *Third Eyes*, August 3rd.

Alubo, S.O., 1990. "State, Violence and Health in Nigeria". *Social Science and Medicine*, 31: 1075-1084.

Anderson, O.W. and J. Foldman, 1956. *Family Medical Insurance: A Nationwide Survey*. New York, McGraw-Hill.

Aregbeyen, M, 1992. *Health Care Service Utilization in Nigeria Rural Communities: A Focus on Otuo Community and its Environment in Ondo State*. Ibadan, NISER.

Aregbeyen, M., 1988. "Public Health Service Finance in Nigeria", *The Economic Insight*. Ile-Ife, Obafemi Awolowo University Press.

Aregbeyen, M., 1991. *Economic Implication of Preventive Health Care: The Case of Environmental Sanitation Board, Ibadan*. NISER Monograph. Ibadan, NISER.

Asakitikpi, A.E., 2005. "Risk Factors and Behavioral Patterns Affecting Childhood Diarrhea in Ibadan. An unpublished PhD thesis in Sociology, University of Ibadan.

Barnett, H.G., 1953. *Innovation: The Basis of Culture Change*. London, McGraw-Hill.

Ben Ami, A., 1969. *Social Change in a Hostile Environment: The Crusaders Kingdoms of Jerusalem*. Princeton, University Press.

Bendix, M., 1967. "Tradition and Modernity Reconsidered", *Comparative Studies of Societies and History*, 2: 57-72.

Benedict Ruth, 1941. "Anthropology and Cultural Change", *American Scholar*, 11: 234-256.

Bennett, F.J., 1986. "Introduction: Health Resolution in Africa", *Social Science and Medicine*, 22 (7): 1052-1064.

Bennis, W. & Bennis, 1974. *The Planning of Change*. London, Holt Rinehart.

Bonsi, K.K., 1977. "Persistence and Change in Traditional Medical Practice in Ghana", *International Journal of Comparative Sociology* 14 (182): 213-245.

Bonsi, K.K., 1979. Becoming a Traditional Healer: Some Similarities and Differences between Western Medicine and Traditional Medical Education". A Monograph of the University of Jos, Nigeria.

Bonsi, K.K., 1980. "Modernization of Native Healers: Implication for Health Care Delivery in Ghana", *Journal of National Medical Association*, 72 (1): 34-56.

Borrisson and Rathwell, 1996. "Health Care Reforms in Bulgaria: An Initial Appraisal, *Social Science and Medicine*, 42 (11): 1023-1045.

Burdillon, M.F.C., 1991. "Religion, Medicine and Healing". In: Olupona J.K. and T. Falola (eds) *Religion and Society in Nigeria: Historical and Sociological Perspective*. London, Routledge, 76-87.

Campbell, M.J. 1990. *New Technology and Rural Development: The Social Impact*. London, Routledge.

Carley, M. and W. Derow, 1984. "Social Impact Assessment: A Cross Disciplinary Guide to the Literature", *Policy Studies*.

Castle, S.E., 1995. "Child Fostering and Children's Nutritional Outcome in Rural Mali: The Role of Female Status in Directing Child Transfer", *Social Science and Medicine*, 40 (5): 765-798.

Clark, A.E., 1990. "Women's Health: Life Cycle Issues". In: R.D. Apple (ed.) *Women, Health and Medicine in America: A Historical Handbook*. New York, Garland, 79-94.

Clark, J.P., 1982. *"Abiku"*, in *West African Verse – An Anthology, Chosen and Annotated by Donatus, Ibe Nwaga* .Longman, United Kingdom.

Coliver, A. et. al., 1967. "Factor Influencing the Use of Maternal Health Services". *Social Science and Medicine*, September: 293-308.

Curtic, L.A., 1975. *Violence, Race and Culture*. Lexington M.A, Lexington Books.

Daramola, O and J. Aina, 1972. *"Asa ati Orisa Ile Yoruba"*. Ibadan, Onibonoje Press.

D'Souza, S., 1989. "The Assessment of Preventable Infant and Child Death in Developing Countries: Some Implications of a New Index" *World Health Statistics Quarterly,* 42: 16-25.

David Landy, 1977. *Culture, Disease and Healing: Studies in Medical Anthropology* .New York, Macmillan.

Desai, B., 1990. "Managing Ecological Upheavals: A Third World Perspective", *Social Science and Medicine,* 30: 1065-1072.

Dreze and Sen, 1990. (Ed.) *The Political Economy of Hunger.* Oxford, Clarendon Press.

Ebrahim, G.J., 1982. *Child Health in Changing Environment.* London, Macmillan.

Egbert, D., 1991. *Man in Rapid Social Change Environment* .London, SCM Press Ltd.

Ember and Ember, 1973. *Anthropology.* New York, Appleton Century Crafts.

Erinosho, O.A., 1977. "Attitudes to Rural Practice among Nigerian Medical Students". *Nigerian Medical Journal,* 7 (4): 472-475.

Erinosho, O.A., 1998. *Health Sociology.* Ibadan, Sam Bookman.

Evans, P and E. Stoddart, 1990. "Producing Health, Consuming Health Care". *Social Science and Medicine,* 31: 1475-1482.

F.O.S., 1998. Bulletin on Population Variables in Osun State (Federal Office of Statistics, Abuja).

Fadipe, N.A., 1970. *The Sociology of the Yorubas.* Ibadan, Ibadan University Press.

Feder, G. and D.L Umali, 1993. "The Adoption of Agricultural Innovations: A Review". *Technology Forecasting and Social Change,* 43: 215-239.

Firth Raymond, 1959. *Social Change in Tukopia.* London, Allen & Unwin.

Fliege, F. 1993. *Diffusion Research in Rural Sociology: The Record and Prospects for the Future* .West Port C.T, Greenwood Press.

Fooster, S.O., 1984. "Intervening Variables and Parasitic Diseases in Child Survival Strategies for Research". *Supplement Population and Development Review,* 10: 130-154.

Grace, J., 1997. "Health Development and Sasak Women: A Political and Practical Analysis of Medical Intervention in East Lumbok, Indonesia", Thesis, Murdock University, Western Australia.

Grace, J., 1997. "The Treatment of Infants and Young Children Suffering Respiratory Tract Infection and Diarrhea Disease in Rural Community in South East Indonesia", *Social Science and Medicine,* 46 (10): 1291-1302.

Harrison Kelsey, 1998. "The Scope of Reproductive Health Research in Africa". *The Network No. 3, March 1998.*

Harry Campbell, 2000. "Strengthening Safe Motherhood" *Child Health Dialogue, Issue 18 (Jan-March): 43-56.*

Holmes, L.D., 1965. *Anthropology: An Introduction.* USA, Roland Press.

House, J.S., Landis, K.R. & Unberson, D. 1988. "Social Relationship and Health", *Science,* 241: 540-545.

Illsley, R., 1950. The Duration of Antenatal Care. *The Medical Officer,* 13: 107-111.

Inkeles, A., 1965. *Becoming Modern.* London, Heinemann.

Isiugo-Abanihe, U and B, Iloh, 1999. "Breastfeeding and its Fertility – Inhibiting Effect in South-Eastern Nigeria", *Journal of Science Research* (Faculty of Science: University of Ibadan) Vol. 5 (1): 4-12.

Jegede, A.S., 1994. *"Aisan" as a Social Term in Nigerian Perspective of Illness.* An Award Winning Paper in the Second Worldwide Competition for Young Sociologists.

Jegede, A.S., 1997. Family Planning Information Sources and Media Exposure among Nigerian Male Adolescents: Case Study of Ekiti South-West Local Government Are of Ondo State. UEPA No. 28, 1997.

Jelliffe, D.B. &F.J Bennett, 1960. "Indigenous Medical Systems and Child Health". *Journal of Peadiatrics,* 57: 248- 256.

Jelliffe, D.B., 1956. "Cultural Variation and the Practical Pediatrician". *Journal of Peadiatrics,* 49: 56-73.

Jelliffe, D.B., 1962. "Culture, Social Change and Infant Feeding: Current Trends in Tropical Regions". *American Journal of Clinical Nutrition,* 10: 67-78.

Jinadu, M.K, 1998. *The Challenge of Health Promotion in Nigeria.* Ile-Ife, Obafemi Awolowo University Press.

Katherine, J.M, 1996. "The Choice of Alternative Therapy for Health Care: Testing Some Propositions", *Social Science and Medicine,* 43 (9): 516-532.

Kelner, M. and P. Wellman, 1997. "Health Care and Consumer Choice: Medical and Alternative Therapies". *Social Science and Medicine,* Vol. 45 (2): 203-212.

Kloss Healmut, 1994. "The Power of Third World: Health and Healthcare in Areas that have yet to Experience Substantial Development". In: David R.P. & V. Yola, (Eds.) *Health and Development.* London, Routledge, 87-106.

Kristen, D.S., 1996. "Maternal and Child Health in Albanja", *Social Science and Medicine,* 43 (7): 947-965.

Lambo, T.A., 1963. *African Traditional Beliefs, Concepts of Health and Medical Practices* .Ibadan, University Press.

Lasker, J.N., 1976 "Health Care and Society in Ivory Coast". An Unpublished PhD Thesis, Harvard University, Cambridge.

Lauer, P. 1973. *Perspective in Social Change* .Boston, Allyne Bacon.

Light, D., 1995. "Equity and Efficiency in Medical Care", *Science and Medicine*, Vol. 35 (4): 465-470.

Linton, R. 1945. "Present World in Cultural Perspective". In: Linton R. (ed.) *The Science of Man in World Crisis*. New York, Columbia University Press, 67-85.

Mabogunje Akin, 2003. "The Real Development Comes From Councils". *Cameroon Tribune*, December 3: 3.

Mark, G.F., 1989. *Success and Crisis in National Health System: A Comparative Approach*. New York, Routledge.

Mehtap Tatar, 1996. "Community Participation in Health Care: The Turkish Care". *Science and Medicine*, 40 (5): 827-845.

Moore, F., 1963. *Social Change*. New York, Prentice Hall Press.

Morely, D. and Lovel, H., 1986. *My Name is Today*. London, Macmillan.

Morgan, L.M., 1993. *Community Participation in Health: The Politics of Primary Health Care in Costa Rica*. New York, Cambridge University Press.

National Population Commission, Nigeria, 2006. Nigerian Population Figure, 2006. Abuja, Federal Ministry of Information.

Nevarro, V., 1974. "The Underdevelopment of Health of Health of Underdevelopment: An Analysis of the Distribution in Latin America". *International Journal of Health Science,* 4 (1): 45- 74.

Odebiyi, A.I., 1977. "Socio-cultural Factors Affecting Health Delivery in n Nigeria". *Journal of Tropical Hygiene* Vol. 80 (11): 248-259.

Odebiyi, A.I., 1999. "Social Factors in Health", Inaugural Lecture Series 136 Delivered at Obafemi Awolowo University, Ile-Ife, Nigeria. Ile-Ife, Obafemi Awolowo University Press.

Ogburn, W.F., 1967. *An Introduction of Sociological Studies*. London, Heinemann.

Ojo, G.J.A., 1966. *The Yoruba Culture*. Oxford, Oxford University Press.

Okafor, S.I., 1982. Spatial Location and Utilization of Health Facilities. In, O.A. Erinosho (Ed.) *Nigerian Perspectives on Medical Sociology. Studies in Third World Societies*, 19: 79-98.

Oke, E.A.,1987. *An Introduction to Social Anthropology*. London, Macmillan.

Oke, E.A., 1993a. "The Essence of PHC in Developing Society: The Nigerian Experience". In: Oke, E.A. and B.E Owumi (Eds) *Primary Health Care in Nigeria State of Art*. Ibadan, Department of Sociology: 34-52.

Oke, E.A.,1993b. "Culture, Man and Utilization Pattern". A Paper Presented at the 2nd Workshop for PHC Officers and Coordinators, Family Planning Officers, Monitoring and Evaluation Officers at the Local Government Level, University of Ibadan, Nigeria, 29-31 March.

Oke, E.A., 1996. "Adaptation of Anthropological Mythodologies to Health Care Delivery Programmes". In: Oke, E.A. and B.E Owumi (Eds.) *Readings in Medical Sociology*. Ibadan, RDMS, 67-85.

Oluwadare, C.T., 2000. "Socio-cultural Factors Influencing Breast Feeding Practice in Ondo State, Nigeria". An unpublished PhD. Thesis in the Department of Sociology, University of Ibadan, Ibadan, Nigeria.

Omorodion, F.I., 1993. "The Socio-cultural Context of Health Behavior among Esan Community, Edo State, Nigeria". *Health Transition Review,* 3 (2): 1312-1150.

Osunwole, S.A., 1989. "Healing in Yoruba Traditional Belief System". An Unpublished PhD. Thesis, Institute of African Studies, University of Ibadan, Ibadan, Nigeria.

Otite, O., 1994. "Social Sciences and Preventive Medicine", *Social Science and Medicine,* 20(10): 876-904.

Otite, O. and Oginowo, 1981. *Introduction to Sociological Studies.* Nigeria, Heinemann.

Owumi, B.E., 1989. "Physician-Patients Relationship in an Alternative Health Care System among the Okpe People of Bendel State". An Unpublished PhD Thesis, Faculty of Social Sciences, University of Ibadan, Ibadan, Nigeria.

Owumi, B.E., 1993. "The Place of Traditional Medicine in PHC". In, Oke, E.A. and B.E Owumi (Eds.) *Primary Health Care State of Art.* Ibadan, Department of Sociology.

Patrick, D.L., Stein, J., Porta, M., Porter, Q. and T.C Ricketts, 1988. *Poverty, Health Services and Health Status: Lessons from Rural America* (Milbank Q), 66: 105-136.

Patrick, P.L. & Wickizer, 1995. "Community and Health". In: Amick, B.J.(Ed.) *Society and Health.* New York, Oxford University Press.

Pearce, T.O. (1986) "Social Change and the Modernization of Medical System". In: Afonja, S and T.O Pearce (Eds) *Social Change in Nigeria.* England, Longman.

Pick and Obermeyer, 1996. "Urbanization, Household Composition and Reproductive Health of Women in South Africa". *Social Science and Medicine* Vol. 43 (10): 1543-1560.

Population Reference Bureau (1995, 1997) World Population Data Sheets, Washington, D.C.

Price Penny, 1994. "Maternal and Child Health Care Strategies". In: David, R.P. and Yola Verhasselt (Eds.) *Health and Development.* London: Routledge, 115-143.

Raikes, A., 1989. "Women Health in East Africa". *Social Science and Medicine,* 28(5): 447-459.

Read, M.,1966. *Culture, Health and Disease.* London, Livestock Publication Ltd.

Richard, W.L. 1974. "Medical Anthropology". In: John, J (Ed) *Handbook of Social and Cultural Anthropology* .Chicago, McNally.

Roemer, M.I., 1991. National Health System of the World, Vol. 1. Oxford, Oxford University Press.

Rosenstock, I.M., 1966. Why People Use Health Services. *Milbank Memorial Fund Quarterly*, 44: 94-127.

Rosenstock, I.M., 1974. Historical Origin of the Health Belief Model. In: Becker M.H. (ed.) *Health Belief Model and Personal Health Behaviour*. Thorofare, N.J. Slack, 1-8.

Rovers, E.M., 1983. *Diffusion of Innovation*. New York, The Press.

Royston, E. and Armstrong, S. (ed.), 1989. *Preventing Maternal Deaths* Geneva, World Health Organization.

Sachs, L. and G. Tomson, 1992. "Medicine and Culture: A Double Perspective on Drug Utilization in a Developing Country". *Social Science and Medicine*, 34 (3): 307-315.

Saginga, C.P., 1998. "An Assessment of Social Impact of Improved Agricultural Technologies: The Case of Soybean Adoption in Benue State, Nigeria". An Unpublished PhD Thesis in the Department of Sociology, University of Ibadan, Ibadan, Nigeria.

Saltman, R., 1989. "Public Competition versus Mixed Market: An Analytical Comparison". *Health Policy II*.

Schram, R., 1971. *A History of the Nigerian Health Services*. Ibadan, University Press.

Sofowora, A.B., 1982. *Medicine, Plants and Traditional Medicine in Africa* New York, John Wiley and Sons Ltd.

Soyinka, Wole,1982. *Abiku, in West Africa Verse: An Anthology, Chosen and Annotated* by Donatus Ibenwogu. United Kingdom, Longman.

Symke, P., 1991. *Women and Health*. London, Zed Books.

Tella, A., 1992. Traditional/Alternative Medicine in Quest of Health for All by the Year 2000A.D. An Inaugural Lecture Series 51, University of Maiduguri, Nigeria. Maiduguri, University Press.

Tim Cullinan, 2000. "Safe Motherhood is Everybody's Business". *Child Health Dialogue*, 18 (January-March): 23-43.

Twaddle, A.C., 1989. "Scandinavian Medical Care and the Crisis in Western Medicine". *Scandinavian Studies*, 61: 217-232.

Twaddle, A.C. 1996. Health System for International Comparison. *Social Science and Medicine*, 43(5): 654-663.

United Nations Children Fund (Annuals 1990-1998) *The State of the World Children*. Oxford, University Press.

Williams, C.D., Bausmalang, N. and D.B, Jelliffe, 1989. *Mother and Child Health: Delivering the Services*. Oxford, University Press.

World Bank, 1991. *World Development Report 1991*. New York, Oxford University Press.

86   Rural Health Provisioning

World Health Organization (Annuals 1960, 1976, 1978, 1991, 1996, 1998 and 2008) *Maternal Health around the World*.

Young, A., 1981. "The Creation of Medical Knowledge: Some Problems in Interpretation". *Social Science and Medicine*, 15 B: 356-379.

Zaidi, S.A., 1988. "Poverty and Disease: Need for Structural Change". *Social Science and Medicine*, 27: 335-365.

Zakus, J.D.I.,1988. "Resources Dependency and Community Participation in Primary Health Care". *Social Science and Medicine*, 46(4-5): 475-494.

Index

Aare 58
Àbíkú 3, 4
Acculturation 11
Ailera 58
Ajaba .... XII, 20, 30, 31, 32, 33, 34
Ajítòní 4
Aladuras 63
Alternative .... IX, XI, 11, 12, 63, 86, 88, 89
Amodi 58
Anti-social 57
Aregbeyen 1, 2, 3, 5, 51, 52, 83
Basic Health Services Scheme 3
Bio-cultural problems 1, 2
Child healthcare IX, 1, 2, 6, 7, 9, 11, 13, 19,
    20, 22, 32, 48, 51, 60, 80, 81, 82
Child rearing 77, 78
Child Survival Initiative 52
Cholera 2, 4, 16, 37, 42, 71, 73
Christ Apostolic Church .... XI, 45, 60, 63
Cultural patterns 9, 54, 77, 78
Cultural prejudices 11
Culture .... VII, XII, XIII, XIV, 1, 2, 5, 8, 9,
    10, 11, 12, 13, 15, 17, 18, 19, 49, 50, 51,
    54, 58, 59, 77, 78, 79, 84, 85, 86, 87, 88,
    89
Culture content .... XIV, 10, 12
Determinants of health 50, 54
Diachronism 9
Diarrhea 4, 37, 65, 66, 73, 74, 83, 85
Diphtheria 4, 71, 73
Disease ...15, 16, 49, 50, 54, 57, 58, 76, 81,
    85, 89, 90
Divine oil 60
Dr. Olikoye Ransome-Kuti 7
Ebrahim 1, 2, 4, 85
Ekusa .... XII, 20, 30, 31, 35, 36, 71, 72
Eléwé-omo 4, 5
Emic 19
Empty-cell family 69
Endogenous 11
Ethnography .... VII, XII, 19, 23, 32
Etic 19
Exogenous 11, 12
Facial tribal mark 26
Faith healing 59
Family income 54
Food discrimination 66

Gender equality 1
Genetricem 30
Health Belief Model . IX, XI, XII, 8, 14, 89
Health education 3, 7, 14, 72, 78, 81
Healthcare organization 50
Holy water 60, 63
Homeostasis 57
Host culture 11
Housing pattern 35, 41
Human biology 50
Ìgbékòyí 4
Ila-Orangun 21, 32, 33, 34
Ilobu 7, 21, 27, 39, 41
Immunization .... XI, 7, 12, 53, 71, 72, 79
Incantation 62
Index 57
Indigestible 66
Inisha 21, 36
Innovation IX, XII, 8, 9, 10, 11, 13, 14, 78,
    84, 89
Integration 5, 11, 13, 59, 78, 81
Intensive breastfeeding 65
Inter-societal contact 10
Interview guides 21
Iyun 1, 5
Jinadu 1, 2, 3, 4, 12, 52, 86
Key informants interview 22, 24
Kwashiorkor 16, 58, 68, 73
Lactate 68
Malaria .... VII, 2, 37, 58, 71, 73
Malnutrition .. 2, 4, 6, 16, 17, 21, 71, 73, 74
Málomó 4
Marasmus 4, 68, 71
Market 29, 32, 34, 36, 38, 43, 44, 45, 89
Maternal V, VII, IX, X, XI, XIII, XIV, 1, 2,
    3, 4, 5, 6, 7, 8, 9, 11, 12, 14, 15, 16, 17,
    18, 19, 20, 22, 23, 24, 31, 32, 48, 49, 51,
    52, 53, 54, 55, 57, 59, 60, 63, 65, 67, 68,
    69, 70, 71, 72, 73, 74, 75, 76, 77, 79, 80,
    81, 82, 83, 84, 86, 89, 90
Maternal and Child Healthcare VII, IX, XI,
    2, 3, 5, 6, 7, 8, 9, 11, 12, 14, 19, 20, 22,
    23, 24, 31, 32, 48, 49, 51, 53, 54, 55, 57,
    59, 60, 63, 65, 69, 71, 72, 73, 77, 80, 82
Maternal and Child Healthcare
    Development Programmes .... XI, 12
Maternity centres 63, 69

Measles 4, 62
Medicine and culture 49, 50
Modern culture 9
Modern medicine....3, 4, 13, 14, 51, 52, 61, 62
Modification 11, 81
Morbidity and mortality VII, IX, X, XIV, 1, 2, 5, 7, 8, 12, 17, 70, 71, 76, 80, 81
Natural and preter-natural explanations 2
Nevarro 1, 87
Observational technique 22, 23
Odebiyi 1, 3, 4, 5, 12, 50, 51, 87
Ògbánje 2
Ojojo 58
Oke .. IX, 1, 5, 9, 32, 34, 38, 49, 50, 53, 87, 88
Okinni... XII, 20, 30, 31, 38, 39, 40, 41, 61, 63, 71, 72
Osogbo 20, 21, 27, 28, 29, 36, 39, 41, 43
Osun State V, VII, IX, XIV, 4, 5, 6, 7, 8, 9, 11, 16, 19, 20, 25, 27, 29, 30, 31, 32, 35, 39, 41, 42, 44, 45, 48, 55, 57, 60, 62, 63, 65, 70, 71, 72, 73, 75, 80, 83, 85
Owumi 1, 3, 4, 5, 50, 51, 52, 87, 88
Pathological abnormality 57
Poliomyelitis 4, 71, 73
Polygyny 12, 29, 34, 63
Prayer 35, 60, 63
Primary Health Care.... XI, 3, 7, 19, 20, 31, 53, 59, 70, 71, 82, 87, 88, 90
Primary Schools 31, 41
Progressive adjustment 11
Random sampling 20, 21
Replacement 11, 12
Resilient 6, 9, 10, 12, 18, 52, 66, 71
Richard 1, 2, 89

Risks of childbearing and child healthcare 1
Royston and Armstrong 1
Rural Health Care VII, XIII, 3, 5, 73, 76, 77
Safe delivery 59
Securing pregnancy 58
Sexual abstinence 65
Smyke 1, 5, 52, 53
Snowball approach 22
Social change 8, 9, 49, 55, 78
Social empowerment 81
Social Impact Assessment ... IX, XI, XII, 8, 13, 84
Socio-demographic characteristics 48
Structured interview .... IX, 21, 22, 23, 24
Sustainable health programme 71
Synchronism 9
Syncretic medicine 63
Syncretism 11, 12, 59, 60, 61, 63
Tetanus 4, 71, 73
Tonkere XIII, 20, 27, 30, 31, 44, 45, 63, 72
Traditional Birth Attendants/pediatricians 4
Traditional culture 9, 20
Traditional healers ... 11, 22, 23, 28, 36, 61, 62, 67
Traditional medicine VII, XIV, 3, 5, 12, 13, 16, 49, 50, 51, 61, 62, 79
Traditional value 18
Traditional Yoruba conception of health 57
Transformatory-integrational model 78
Typhoid 4, 37
UNICEF .... XI, 1, 2, 6, 46, 52
Uxorem 30
Weaving 28, 37
World Health Organization.... XI, 1, 57, 89, 90
Yoruba rural communities 2

www.ingramcontent.com/pod-product-compliance
Lightning Source LLC
Chambersburg PA
CBHW070756300326

41914CB00053B/686